Cannabis for Canines

Beverly A. Potter, Ph.D.

"Docpotter"

RONIN

Berkeley, California

Important Notice:

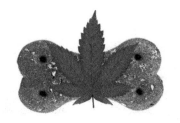

Cannabis for Canines

Beverly A. Potter, Ph.D.

"Docpotter"

Cannabis for Canines

Published by

Ronin Publishing, Inc.

PO Box 3436

Oakland, CA 94609

www.roninpub.com

Production:

    Manuscript Creaton: Beverly A. Potter, Ph.D.

    Cover Design: bgdesign09@gmail.com

    Book Design: Beverly A. Potter.

    Content Creation: Abby Hauck/CannabisContent.com

    Photos: Fotolia, Pixabay

Library of Congress Card Number: 2018949372

Manufactured in the United States by **Lightning Source**.

Distributed to the book trade by **PGW/Ingram**.

Acknowledgements

Thank you, Dear Readers, for picking up this book. May you find inspiration and comfort for your beloved dog in the information shared here in.

A special thanks to Abby Hauck of Cannabis Content for her help in preparing the manuscript; to veterinarian Dr. Gary Richter for his bravely providing solid dosing information to dog owners under his right to free speech, to Green Camp for their infographic, to King Kanine, Canna-Pet and HolistaPet for their great products and useful educational information, to Blake Armstrong for his leadership and helpful reviews, to Green-Flower for their excellent educational programs. Thank you all for your ground-breaking work and invaluable contributions to *Cannabis for Canines.*

—Docpotter

Books by Docpotter

- **Cannabis for Seniors**

- **The Healing Magic of Cannabis**
It's the High that Heals!

- **Marijuana Recipies & Remedies for Healthy Living**
as Mary Jane Stawell

- **Overcoming Job Burnout:**
How To Renew Enthusiasm For Work

- **Finding A Path With A Heart**
How To Go From Burnout To Bliss

- **The Worrywart's Companion**
21 Ways to Soothe Yourself & Worry Smart

- **From Conflict To Cooperation:**
How To Mediate A Dispute

- **Get Peak Performance Every Day**
How to Manage Like a Coach

- **High Performance Goal Setting**
Using Intuition to Conceive & Achieve Your Dreams

- **Brain Boosters**
Foods & Drugs That Make You Smarter

- **Heal Yourself**
Turn on the Power of Placebo

- **Drug Testing At Work**
A Guide For Employers And Employees

- **Pass the Test**
An Employee Guide to Drug Testing

- **The Way Of The Ronin**
Riding The Waves Of Change At Work

- **Turning Around**
Keys To Motivation & Productivity

- **Preventing Job Burnout:**
A Workbook

- **Youth Extension A-Z**

- **Beyond Consciousness:**
What Happens After Death

- **Patriots Handbook**

- **Spiritual Secrets for Playing the Game of Life**

- **Simple Pleasures**

- **Question Authority to Think for Yourself**

- **Managing Yourself for Excellence**
How to Become a Can-Do Person

- **Healing Hormones**
How to Turn On Natural Chemicals to Reduce Stress

Table of Contents

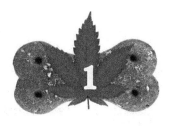

Introduction

Dogs are cherished family members. Just as we want the best for our parents, siblings, and children, we want the best for our beloved family dogs. Whether your dog has eating upsets, anxiety, lethargy, cancer, seizures, or another aliment, you've likely heard that cannabis supplements can support your vet's treatment—and possibly be an alternative to using strong pharmaceuticals. The answer is "yes, but!".

Unfortunately, because cannabis was criminalized by *Marijuana Tax Act in 1937* and then later classified in 1970 as a Schedule 1 "drug" under the federal Controlled Substance Act, there has been little research

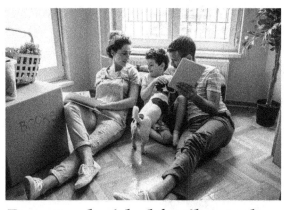

Dogs are cherished family members

The American Holistic Veterinary Medical Association [AHVMA] is the first veterinary organization to officially encourage research into the use of cannabis for animals.

for decades. Worse, as you will learn in the following pages, while "medical marijuana" has been legalized in many States, none of the State bills included dogs. In fact, veterinarians who prescribe or sell cannabis—in any form—risk losing their license. Fortunately, there are pressures to reform this "retrograde" policy.

The American Holistic Veterinary Medical Association [AHVMA] is the first veterinary organization to officially encourage research into the use of cannabis for animals. They said, "There is a growing body of veterinary evidence that cannabis can reduce pain and nausea in chronically ill or suffering animals, often without the dulling effects of narcotics. This herb may be able to improve the quality of life for many patients, even in the face of life-threatening illnesses." This should make dog "parents" take notice.

The Aussies took the lead when in February 2016, Australia legalized medicinal cannabis at its federal level. Dr. Edward Bassingthwaighte, an Australian holistic vet, told *Dogs Naturally Magazine* that "medical cannabis has few adverse side effects, as long as you don't overdose." That is encouraging but is a little like saying, "flying is great, so long as you don't crash."

Endocannabinoid System

Cannabinoids, chemicals in cannabis, accomplish their beneficial effects by way of the Endocannabinoid System [ECS]—comprised by a multitude of cannabinoid receptor sites located throughout our bodies and those of our dogs. As you will learn in the following pages, when a cannabinoid, like Cannabidiol [CBD], as an example, plugs into receptors in the ECS beneficial effects are turned on or negative effects tuned off.

Scientists believe that the purpose of the EC system to whole body homeostasis.

Using Cannabis

Cannabis offers a multitude of health benefits for both humans and canines. Because receptor sites in the ECS are located throughout the body, including the skin, muscles, brain, nerves, and immune system, cannabis therapeutics can beneficially impact a broad range of bodily systems.

• **Digestive Upsets**—Dog digestive systems are more sensitive than those of humans, which is surprising considering that dogs love to chew and may attempt to eat just about anything. Dogs can have digestive issues, including sensitive stomach, irritable bowels, diarrhea, vomiting, and gastritis, which is chronic inflammation of the stomach.

• **Anxiety and Phobias**—Many dogs "freak out" when left home alone, called separation anxiety. Major events like the death of a companion dog or moving to a new home can cause a well-adjusted dog to become anxious. Loud noises like fireworks is a common anxiety trigger. Such stressful events may lead to destructive behavior, like chewing shoes and furniture, and negative reactions, like howling when alone as well as growling and snapping.

• **Arthritis and Joint Stiffness** —Signs of joint disease include stiffness, limping, or favoring a limb—particularly after resting, inability to rise, jump, or climb stairs, often with noticeable pain. Aging dogs, especially large breeds, often develop arthritis as a result of years of wear and tear on joints and ligaments, so they struggle with getting up, climbing stairs, and jumping and onto the bed for hugs.

• **Skin and Coat**—Many dogs scratch and chew themselves excessively, creating "hot spots" because of skin issues, including allergies, dermatitis, mange, and flea infestations.

• **Malaise and Lethargy**—A healthy immune system identifies potentially harmful pathogens like bacteria, viruses, fungi, and parasites, and eliminates them before they can do harm. When the immune system is compromised, your dog becomes vulnerable to illness. A malfunctioning immune system can open the door to infections and diseases.

• **Epilepsy and Seizures**—Epilepsy is probably the most well-known neurological disorder in dogs, characterized by recurrent seizures. Dogs may suffer seizures as a result of eating poison, a head injury or a disease.

• **Heart and Circulatory Issues**—Dogs can suffer heart and circulatory problems, such as congestive heart failure, heartworm disease.

• **Pain and Inflammation**—Pain can be caused by a wide range of problems, from toothaches to arthritis to pancreatitis. The swelling that accompanies inflammation generally causes pain as it pushes against sensitive nerve endings that send pain signals to the brain.

• **Cancer**—Cancer is the leading cause of death in dogs over 2 years of age. Vets tend to focus treatment on symptom management with the goal of reducing pain and suffering, rather than life extension.

Promising Alternative

Cannabis offers a safe, low-impact benefit to symptoms of many conditions as well as for side effects of many pharmaceutical medications. Cannabis derivatives can increase appetite and energy levels, help speed recovery time, as well as offering much-need relief from pain and spasms along with reducing anxiety and aggression, among other benefits.

Medicinal cannabis is an emerging veterarian specialty. Dosing is a challenge and is very different for small animals, as compared with for humans.

Cannabis is best used as a suppliment—a helpful component of a health plan tailored to your dog, rather than as a sole treatment. Keep your vet in the loop.

Family Health

Dogs have a big impact upon our well-being. Seeing, touching, hearing and talking to our beloved dogs releases, beneficial neurohormones that induce a wonderful sense of goodwill, joy, nurturing and happiness. At the same time, the stress hormone cortisol is suppressed. Heart rate, blood pressure and respiratory rate can all decrease, leaving us more relaxed.

Thanks BFF!!!

[Best Friends Forever!!!]

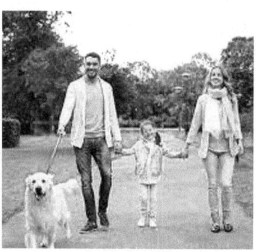

A happy, healthy family.

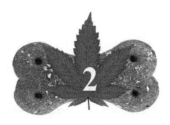

Veterinary Meds

When your dog is sick, injured or anxious, your vet may prescribe a medication. Some medications are available over-the-counter, while other drugs that may be more complicated to administer or those prone to interacting with other medications will always require a veterinarian's prescription. Preventative heartworm medication, for example, is prescribed to dogs who do not already have heartworm because the preven-

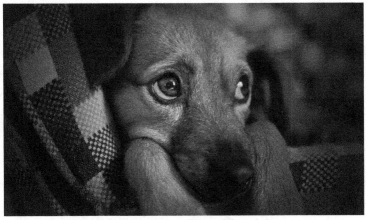

Keep your dog-friend healthy.

tative medicines attack larva but not the adult heartworm. In some cases, heartworm-positive dogs taking preventative heartworm medication may develop a potentially deadly anaphylactic reaction when the drug attacks too many larva at a time. To prevent such tragedies, obtaining a prescription heartworm medication from a veterinarian is imperative.

Vets may prescribe medications when the dosing instructions are precise or complicated. Spot-on flea and tick medication, for example, must be used exactly as instructed and for only for the type of animal for which it is manufactured. It's not that the drug is exceptionally potent or otherwise dangerous, necessarily, just that the drug manufacturer and veterinarians have decided that one-on-one instructions on how to use the product should be included in the purchase of the drug itself in order for it to be effective.

Antibiotics

Antibiotics—or antibacterial—are an antimicrobial drug used to treat or prevent bacterial infections. They are used to kill existing bacteria or to stop it from replicating and spreading throughout the body. Antibiotics may be prescribed after an injury or surgery to reduce the risk of infection, or they can be used retroactively after an infection has taken hold to treat conditions like gastrointestinal, respiratory, ear or skin infections.

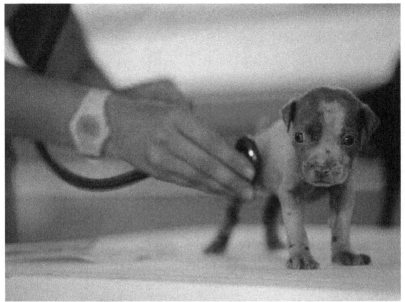

Puppy being examined by vet.

Antibiotics are generally an effective way to prevent or stop the spread of bacteria-related infections, but some bacteria can become resistant to antibiotics—which is especially likely when previously-prescribed antibiotics like penicillin were not finished before cessation—making infection more dangerous and even life-threatening in some cases.

Antibiotics, like penicillin or amoxicillin, can have adverse consequences when misused. Because there are a variety of antibiotics with different applications, the veterinarian must assess your dog's specific needs and prescribe the appropriate antimicrobial drug accordingly along with precise dosing instructions. A vet must be careful to not prescribe medicine intended to reduce fungal infections if the infection is bacterial, for example.

If a dog takes the wrong antibiotic or you do not follow dosing instructions carefully, the medication may not sufficiently stop the spread of the infection thus encouraging your dog to developed a tolerance to the antibiotic due to you having given a too low dose so it may return with a vengeance. When a veterinarian instructs you to give your dog a specific dose at a specific interval for a specific period, follow the instructions carefully or you risk more significant complications down the road.

Overuse of antibiotics to treat bacterial infection has spawned a treatment-resistant bacteria collectively called *methicillin-resistant Staph aureus* or MSRAs—a.k.a. "superbugs". When dogs contract MSRAs, vets typically prescribe Vancomycin, one of the strongest antibiotics available, but even it can be ineffective at times because of "resistance".

Interestingly, cannabis is showing promise to effectively treat MRSA as well as—or even better—as Vancomycin without increasing the risk of antibiotic resistance. According to a study published in the *US National Library of Medicine*, all five major cannabinoids have shown 'potent activity' against numerous types of treatment-resistant Staph infections. Though we have yet to learn *how* cannabinoids fight against MRSAs, the potential for cannabis to both treat MRSAs and reduce their occurrence is promising.

Non-Steroid Anti-Inflammatory Drugs

NSAIDs are anti-inflammatory drugs prescribed to treat pain and inflamation in ailments like arthritis or swelling after an injury. They work by inhibiting the production of prostaglandins, a hormone-like chemical in the body responsible for regulating inflammatory responses at the site of damage.

Many NSAIDs are available over-the-counter because they are considered relatively safe to consume and easy to administer. However, NSAIDs have risks, including gastrointestinal inflammation and bleeding, which are more likely in older dogs or those taking prescription-strength NSAIDs.

There are many applications for steroid medication including anti-inflammation and immuno-suppression, as well as to reduce aller-

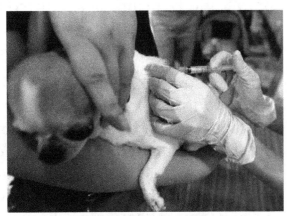

Dog getting a shot.

gic reactions, which can sometimes be fatal. There are many types of steroids that may be prescribed, each intended to mimic the body's own steroid-like chemicals. The two most common types of naturally-occurring steroids include mineralocorticoids—which regulates functions like sodium, chloride and potassium levels in the body as well as blood volume and pressure, and glucocorticoids—which regulate metabolism, development, glucose levels and inflammatory reactions.

Taking high doses of NSAIDs can be life threatening in humans. So it's important to monitor your dog's health and demeanor closely when giving it NSAIDs. Vomiting, diarrhea, loss of appetite and lethargy are symptoms of NSAID toxicity and can be fatal if not addressed properly. Contact your veterinarian if your dog shows these symptoms.

Long-term steroid use—especially in high, immunosuppressive doses—could result in further complications including a reduced ability to heal after injury, urinary tract infections, obesity, muscle weakness and various types of skin infections.

The good news is, cannabis can be used in conjunction with NSAIDs to improve their efficiency and reduce the likelihood of developing unfavorable side effects. According to a study published in the *European Journal of Pharmacology*, low doses of cannabinoids protect "against diclofenac-induced gastric inflammatory tissue damage at doses insufficient to cause common cannabinoid side effects". In other words, the regular use of cannabinoids like CBD protect your dog's gastric track from damage caused by NSAIDs.

Steroids are often required for organ transplantation to be successful as a means of preventing the body from attacking and rejecting the new tissue. High doses of steroids cause an immunosuppressive response in the body, which basically slows the body's own immune responses down while the body adjusts to the new organ. However, extended use of high-dose steroids can cause the body to have difficulty fighting infections later.

Cannabis can effectively reduce immune responses to improve transplant success in animals. According to a study published in the *Journal of Neuroimmune Pharmacology*, "T-cell function was decreased by the CB2 agonists (CBD)…[and] IL-2 release was significantly decreased in the cannabinoid treated cells. Together, these data support the potential of this class of compounds as useful therapies to prolong graft survival in transplant patients"

Opioid Pain Relievers

Opioids are one of the most effective forms of pain relief veterinarians can prescribe. Opioids are used to treat both acute—short term—and chronic—long-lasting—pain by regulating the presynaptic release and postsynaptic response to excitatory neurotransmitters. But opioids come

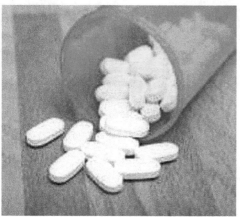

Opioids come with complicaitons.

with complications. For example, some powerful opioids, such as those used during surgery, can cause nausea and respiratory depression, with no ceiling to its effectiveness—the effects increase as the dose increases.

Administration of pure mu-opioid agonists—weakened opioids—must be carefully monitored at all times.Veterinarians may prescribe partial mu-opioid agonists for home administration because they have a significantly lower risk for adverse side effects—although they still exist. So you must be on the alert for symptoms like excessive lethargy, nausea, difficulty breathing or dysphoria.

While such weakened opioids can effectively control pain, they can be difficult to administer, and they take longer to take effect, which means your pooch may be in pain longer than necessary. Dogs cannot communicate their discomfort—and may even instinctively hide it as a survival mechanism, it is important to monitor your dog's demeanor when it is taking opioid pain meds. Vet prescribed opioid pain medication is considered relatively safe for dogs. Some vets, however, are reluctant to prescribe opioids if there's a possibiloity that the dog's owner many be opioid-addicted. For this reason, most vets insist on seeing the dog to assess its needs prior to writing opioid prescriptions.

Antiphrastic Drugs

Antiphrastic drugs are intended to prevent or kill parasites like fleas, ticks or heartworm, and may be administered orally, intravenously or topically. They have been shown to be effective at stopping the spread of parasites provided that the drug being used is targeting the appropriate parasite, and may be administered at home or at the vet's office.

Because we humans are susceptible to parasitic infestation, discuss possible contamination with your vet to determine if further testing is required and to learn proper preventative tactics to avoid your contracting the parasite.

Adding to cannabis's long list of benefits is its use as an antiparasitic. Though there is too little research to say for certain, one study found that members of the Aka tribe in the Congo Ba- ⌐in were significantly less likely to develop intestinal parasites when they consume cannabis.

In fact, people have been using cannabis to help treat and prevent parasites for centuries, dating back to ancient China when cannabis leaves and seeds, dense with non-psychoactive cannabinoids, were juiced and consumed to expel parasites and their larva from the body. The practice has been successfully carried out for many generations since, though we don't quite understand why.

One theory has it that parasites have endocannabinoid systems of their own and are therefore strongly-affected by CBD chemicals that render them infertile and unable to reproduce.

Another theory points to terpenes in the cannabis plant. Terpenes are the aromatic oils that give cannabis and other plants their unique odor and flavor. Terpenes such as limonene, pinene and linalool have antiparasitic properties and may therefore play a role in cannabis's ability to fight parasitic infestation. It is unknown if cannabis deters fleas.

Sedatives

Sedatives are commonly used for anxious dogs to help them to relax or when transported in a crate in the belly of an airplane, as examples. They may also be used to minimize movement during delicate procedures or to prepare for anesthesia.

Prescription sedatives may be administered orally in pill form or by squirting it between the gum and lip for sublingual absorption and may result in a range of effects ranging from seemingly nothing to flat-out lethargy depending on the size, breed, medicinal interactions and so on. It should not come as a surprise that cannabis can alter your dog's mood and demeanor. THC is commonly referenced for it's sedative—or, in some cases, uplifting—effects and can effectively treat anxiety issues like PTSD in humans. It makes sense that cannabis works the same for dogs, as well.

However, THC is a very powerful chemical and could lead to extreme cases of lethargy—rendering your dog completely immobile for a brief period, which may exacerbate its anxiety. Consult a knowledgeable vet before giving your dog THC.

Chemotherapeutics

Cancer is a devastating disease, wreaking havoc on the body—accompanied by terrible pain. The speed at which cancer takes over a dog's body is upsetting. The cost of chemotherapeutic drugs coupled with an already short lifespan prompts most dog owners to choose an alternate route to

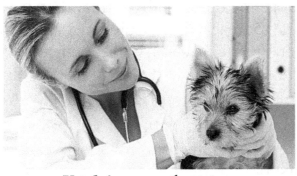

Vet doing exam for cancer.

cancer treatment for their loved canine friend—to help them to be as comfortable as possible for as long as possible.

Most often, canine cancer treatment involves the regular administration of opioid pain relievers. Though these have proven effective for short-term use, long-term opioid consumption can lead to tolerance causing more of the drug to be needed or—because Fido can't talk to you—that your dog suffers needlessly due to ineffective medication and/or dosing.

Condition-Specific Medications

Your veterinarian may prescribe drugs that are specific to certain conditions. For example, a typical occurrence in medium- to large-sized spayed females is a condition called urethral sphincter mechanism incompetence, or USMI, and can be treated successfully with hormone replacement therapy.

Other common condition-specific drugs for dogs include insulin to treat diabetes, levothyroxine to treat hypothyroidism, or trilostane to treat Cushing's disease. These medications tend to be taken life-long and require regular blood work to ensure the dog stays healthy while on medication.

Though the nature of treatment will largely depend on the condition itself, cannabis's long list of therapeutic benefits could help treat multiple problems at once—without over-dosing your pooch with pharmaceutical drugs. For example, cannabis helps reduce pain, increase energy, *Cannabis's broad range of therapeutic benefits may help treat multiple problems at once— without over-dosing your pooch with pharmaceutical drugs.* speed metabolism, reduce anxiety, and prevent bone loss or other hormone-related deficiencies.

Always pay close attention to your dog's behavior and consult your vet when seeing irregularities. Regular cannabis use can help keep your dog healthy and happy, as well as reducing anxiety-causing vet visits, too.

Drug Interactions

Drug interactions are another significant factor determining which medications vets prescribe. Some medicines, for example, may speed or slow metabolism, which can lead to toxicity—if another drug isn't expelled from the body sufficiently, or inef-

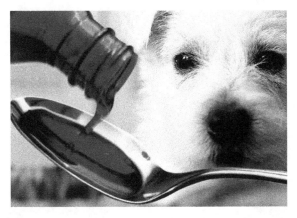

Follow your vet's instructions carefully when giving your dog prescribed drugs

ficiency if too little of the medicine remains in the system long enough to work. While research on human drug interactions has been relatively thorough, canine drug interactions have not been studied as carefully, which highlights the importance of monitoring your dog's reaction while taking a prescription medical regimen.

Maintaining regular veterinary appointments—and carefully following the doctor's orders—is an essential part of ensuring your dog's long-term health, particularly when strong pharmaceuticals are included in treatment

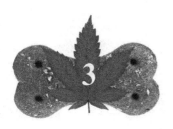

Cannabis Therapeutics

It can be difficult to know when your dog is uncomfortable or even suffering. After all, your dog can't call out, "Hey, Mom, my tommy is aching!" Instead your beloved pooch curls up in its bed while you have your nose in your smart phone, thinking all is well when it may not be so.

For example, I occasionally put my wonderful tan pit, Zoe, in the hot tub, which I did one afternoon. Good that I did because I then noticed a small drop of blood in her nose. "Huh?" I thought and wiped it away with a tissue. It was a Sunday and there's a drop-in vet hospital down the street. So off we went to see the vet. After waiting for nearly two hours, I was telling myself there wasn't really a problem and was about to leave, when the vet called us in for the exam.

Well, it was a medical emergency!!! OMG! Zoe was bleeding internally. Her belly had huge red blotches. I had to get her to the emergency

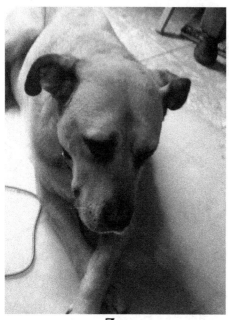

Zoe

vet across town immediately. Off we went, with me driving fast and somewhat reck- lessly, passing cars on the right while hitting the horn, driving over curbs, zooming faster to race through yel- low lights.

The emergency vet explained that Zoe had lost her blood platelets, possibly due to a recent rabies shot. Yes, rabies shots *can* kill. "They" don't tell us this. I lost my favorite cat, Ninja, to a rabies shot!

When I left Zoe that day, the vet couldn't tell me if she would be alive in the morning or if she would "bleed out"! Thankfully, Zoe did survive. When I picked her up her entire belly was a bight red blood blister. She was in and out of the emer- gency vet for check ups for 6 months. The vet gave me a note for Alameda County that exempted Zoe from ever having to have another rabies shot!!!!

Had I *not* noticed that drop of blood on Zoe's nose, she would have gone to her bed and me to the computer—and I likely would have found her dead a few hours later!!!! Thankfully I was fortunate to enjoy 6 more years with my wonderful Zoe.

Cannabis Therapy

Cannabis therapy—the administration of cannabis and cannabis-based potions to benefit over-all health and well-being, has been used by humans for centuries to treat an array of ailments. Stands to reason that dogs can benefit from cannabis, too. However, how cannabis interacts with canines is not fully understood. Giving cannabis to your dog should be entered into with extra precautions to ensure Fido feels better as a result of cannabis therapy and that you don't over do it.

Cannabis offers a long list of health benefits for both humans and canines. However, cannabis can have a more pronounced impact on dogs than it does on us humans. Stress caused by improper dosing, for example, can make your dog uncomfortable or even lethargic, which can lead to numerous complications.

Having said that, there are many benefits of cannabis therapy for canines. The all-natural chemicals derived from cannabis offer a low-impact solution to the symptoms of many conditions as well as for side effects of vet-prescribed medications. It is believed that this is

Consult your vet about your plan and what you hope to accomplish before introducing cannabis into your dog's routine.

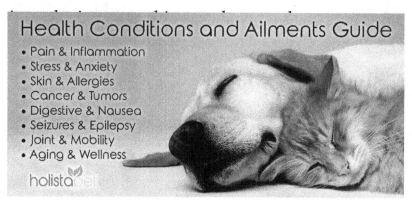

Health Conditions and Ailments Guide
- Pain & Inflammation
- Stress & Anxiety
- Skin & Allergies
- Cancer & Tumors
- Digestive & Nausea
- Seizures & Epilepsy
- Joint & Mobility
- Aging & Wellness

holista

Holistapet offers helpful dog ailment guides on their site.

because cannabinoids resemble chemicals natural-ly produced in the canine body. Cannabis deriva-tives can increase appetite and energy levels, help speed recovery time, as well as offering much-need relief from pain and spasms along with re-ducing anxiety and aggression.

Cannabis therapeutics can be introduced at any time during your dog's life. In addition to sooth-ing pain and nausea, daily cannabis use can help improve your dog's demeanor and stave off many age-related conditions, like bone loss and hormone issues. A dog acting lethargic, refusing to eat, or licking itself excessively may benefit from cannabis therapy.

Likewise, if your dog is to undergo medical treatment by a veterinarian, adding cannabis supplements to its diet may be beneficial. Discuss your plan with the vet before introducing canna-bis into your dog's routine.

Side Effects of CBD in Dogs

• **Dry Mouth:** In humans, CBD affects production of saliva. For dogs, this side effect manifests as increased thirst.

• **Lowering Blood Pressure:** High doses of CBD may cause a drop in blood pressure, causing a temporary feeling of light-headedness.

• **Drowsiness:** The most noticeable effect is a slight drowsiness when high doses of CBD are administered.

• **Inhibition of Drug Metabolism:** High doses of CBD can inhibit or improve the production of some liver enzymes, which may interfere with the metabolism of some drugs.

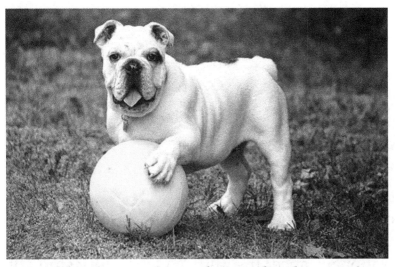

Cannabis therapeutics can be introduced at any time.

Cannabis and Prescription Drugs

Addition of cannabinoids to treatment plan may improve [or inhibit] the effectiveness of many doctor-prescribed medications—as well as over-the-counter [OTC] meds, and can be easily administered at home. Alway check with your vet if your dog is taking a prescription medicine. Here are some of the amazing ways cannabis can assist veterinary-prescribed medications in your dog.

Adding Cannabis to a Dog's Diet

- Dog will be pain-free much longer due to cannabis's analgesic qualities;

- Dog is less likely to develop a tolerance to opioid medication, which helps them maintain their effectiveness;

- Dog's appetite will improve, keeping its energy levels up and helping it fight the ailment;

- Cancer may go into remission.

Cancer Inhibition

Research shows that cannabinoids can stop cancerous tumors from growing and spreading by causing cancer cell death and blocking blood vessels needed to help it spread. According to the National Cancer Institute, "A laboratory study of cannabidiol (CBD) in estrogen receptor positive and estrogen receptor negative breast cancer cells

showed that it caused
cancer cell death while
having little effect on
normal breast cells.

*Cannabinoids may improve
the efficiency of doctor-
prescribed medications*

Studies in mouse models of metastatic breast
cancer showed that cannabinoids may lessen the
growth, number, and spread of tumors. Furthermore, "a review of 34 studies of cannabinoids in
glioma tumor models found that all but one study
showed that cannabinoids can kill cancer cells
without harming normal cells" indicating that numerous types of cancer can be treated with cannabinoids.

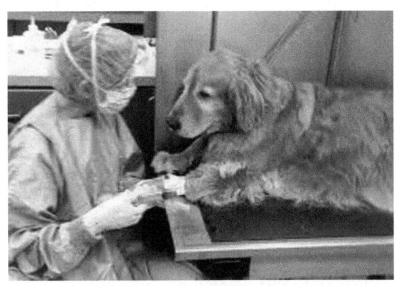

*Many dog owners choose cannabis for their dogs with
cancer not as a cure but as a palliative to help them be
as comfortable as possible.*

Cautions

Cannabis can be a great addition to your dog's medicinal regimen; but effects can be more pronounced in their smaller bodies. Prior to introducing cannabis into your dog's routine, consult your vet about what you hope to accomplish. Though it is likely your vet will not be able to recommend cannabis per se due to licensing laws and lack of research, he or she will likely want to monitor your dog's progress along the way, not only to keep Fido on the path to better health, but also to gain a better understanding of cannabis therapy for their own practice.

When including cannabis into a prescription medical routine, observe your dog's demeanor closely and record everything, good or bad, into a journal. Note the dose, the time, and the frequency of cannabis administration, as well as noticeable changes in your dog's behavior. If anything odd or unsettling occurs, cease cannabis treatment immediately and consult your veterinarian.

Medical advancements have made it possible for dogs to lead longer, happier lives than ever before. Ironically, one of the best forms of therapy may actually be something humans have been using medicinally for centuries, though we're just barely beginning to understand the many benefits. While research is still young, what we've learned so far about cannabinoids has been impressive.

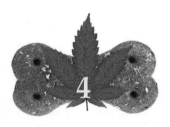

The Endocannabinoid System

The endocannabinoid (EC) system is a collection of cell receptors found throughout our bodies—and those of our dogs. Cell receptors are likened to locks on the surface of certain cells. Chemical messengers, called neurotransmitters, act like a kind of key that fits into and opens the lock, which then relays a message to begin or stop certain processes.

The discovery of the endocannabinoid system began with the isolation of the chemical *Tetrahydrocannabinol*—THC, in 1964 by an Israeli scientist named Raphael Mechoulam. In the 1990s, THC was discovered to exert its effects by binding with special receptors in the brain. Subsequently, scientists discovered more receptors throughout the body and found that endogenous chemicals also interacted with the same receptors. The discovery of the endocannabinoid system

The purpose of the endocannabinoid system seems to be whole body homeostasis.

was named after the cannabis plant that aided in its discovery.

Researchers are working to uncover how cannabinoids exert such a wide range of therapeutic benefits with such minimal risk.

Mitochondria Interaction

In 2012, CB receptors were found to be plentiful in the membranes of mitochondria—the powerhouse of the cell. Because mitochondrial activity plays a major role in cell functionality, the presence of cannabinoid receptors in mitochondria suggests that cannabinoids play a major role in the regulation of inter- as well as intra-cellular communication.

Mitochondria are involved in the regulation of many biological pathways: Neurotransmis-

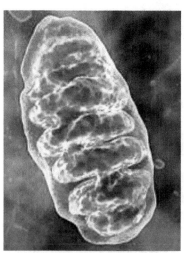

Mitochondria is the powerhouse of the cell.

sion, energy homeostasis and oxidative stress are regulated with cannabinoids. How this happens depends on the cannabinoid and the location of the receptor. For THC to activate mitochondrial cannabinoid receptors, it must first penetrate the cell wall and be ushered into the mitochondria via the surrounding fatty cell membrane. Preclinical

research suggests that
this process can be
beneficial because it
protects the cell from
oxidized stress and
unnecessary apop-
tosis—cell death,
but only at the prop-
er dose. Excessive THC consumption has been
shown to exert the opposite effect, inducing cell
apoptosis—in some circumstances.

*Think of (endocannabinoids)
as being great emcees. They
promote the party, approve the
playlist, get everyone on the
dance floor and wind them all
down at the end of the night.*

—Dr. Tracy E. Foose
Mill Valley Psychiatrist

By contrast, *cannabidiol* (CBD) interacts with
the mitochondria by way of a different set of
receptors located on the mitochondrial surface.
One such receptor, the sodium-calcium exchanger
(NCX), opens an ion channel allowing electrical-
ly-charged ions to either enter into or out of the
cell wall thereby facilitating cellular homeostasis
and neuroprotection.

Both endo—inbody-produced—and phyto—
plant-based—cannabinoids can regulate mitochondrial activity to create a sort of ebb and flow
of calcium deposits to maintain balance, which is
one reason cannabinoids have been shown to protect against brain injury and reduce the likelihood
of developing degenerative brain diseases like
dementia and Alzheimer's. Additionally, cannabinoids have been shown to help protect against
heart attack and stroke by way of the same mechanism.

Need for the Endocannabinoid System

The endocannabinoid system is an integral part of the dog's evolutionary survival. By acting on cells throughout the body and the energy-regulating mitochondria therein, the endocannabinoid system mediates many of the dogs' most primal biological responses.

The EC system regulates a multitude of functions by creating cannabinoids on demand. These endocannabinoids facilitate cellular communication by attaching to receptors on cell walls. They send the information to the inside of the cell to elicit the proper response or action. Sometimes, the action may be to quiet overactive neurons, other times it may be to reduce inflammation.

Because the body produces endocannabinoids as needed then destroys them when no longer needed, no lingering endocannabinoids are stored within the body. Whereas deficiency in endocannabinoid production or overactive endocannabinoid metabolism can lead to chronic conditions like anxiety, fibromyalgia, IBS, and migraines.

Endocannabinoid Supplementation

Humans and dogs as well as all other mammals have an endocannabinoid system. Unfortunately there has been little research on the use of cannabinoids with canines. So we must extrapolate from effects in human.

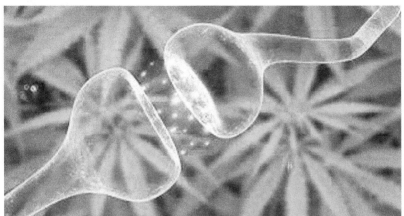

The endocannabinoid system mediates many of the dog's most primal biological responses.

Cannabinoids Help Regulate

- Sleep
- Appetite and Digestion
- Mood
- Motor Control
- Immune function
- Reproduction
- Pain
- Memory
- Body Temperature

Dr. Ethan Russo made an interesting observation in 2001. While seemingly unrelated, many diseases have a few things in common. First, the pain is inexplicable because there is no tissue damage causing it, which points to a biochemical reaction as the cause. Second, these diseases tend to either occur together or to increase the likelihood of developing one after being diagnosed with another. Russo proposed that these conditions could be related to an endocannabinoid deficiency, which theoretically contributes to neurotransmitter deficiencies

Since the publication of Russo's Theory, ample research has been conducted to test it in humans, with positive results. For example, Italian researchers Sarchielli, et al., found in 2007 that chronic migraine sufferers had significantly lower levels of anandamide in their spinal fluid than control subjects. In 2008, researchers Filippo, et al., found the same to be the case among multiple sclerosis patients. The trend continues for conditions like neonatal development, phantom limb pain, infant colic, glaucoma, repetitive miscarriages, post-traumatic stress disorder, bipolar disorder and more.

The enzyme, fatty acid amide hydrolase (FAAH), metabolizes anandamide, which regulates processes like hunger, pain, mood, and so on. When the FAAH enzyme is too active, however, anandamide levels drop, resulting in depressed body functions relating to the endocannabinoid system. Because low levels of anandamide can cause malfunctions throughout the body, it stands to reason that supplementation with either synthetic or phytocannabinoids may help correct the discrepancy. Research shows that

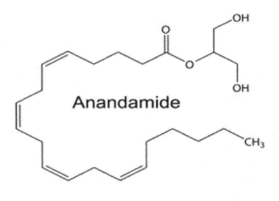

Anandamide

CBD does so and in a very interesting way.

Research suggests that phytocannabinoid supplementation—specifically, THC—is beneficial only to a certain extent, at which point its therapeutic benefits begin to taper off, which is one reason THC tends to relax some people while making others anxious.

By contrast, CBD functions differently. Unlike THC, which binds to the same receptors as does anandamide and other endocannabinoids, CBD acts as an antagonist, blocking CB receptors and controlling their flow. CBD can inhibit the release of the FAAH enzyme, thus improving the concentration of anandamide throughout the body. Essentially, CBD supplementation can help boost your dog's internal endocannabinoid production, slow its metabolism, and thus improve deficiencies in endocannabinoid system functioning.

Sources of Cannabinoids

Anandamide and 2-Arachidonoylglycerol (2-AG) are two of the most common endocannabinoids that regulate sleep, appetite, pain perception and other processes. Synthetic cannabinoids also interact with the endocannabinoid system. Importantly, synthetic cannabinoids should be approved by a vet because some are not fit for consumption. In fact, some synthetic cannabinoids sold on the black market are dangerous because they fully bind to CB receptors.

There are phytocannabinoids, which come from plants. While the cannabis plant is an excellent source of cannabinoids, it's not the only source! Though cannabis-derived cannabinoids seem to be the only ones that interact with CB1 receptors that elicit psychoactive qualities, others interact with CB2 receptors in peripheral tissue throughout the rest of the body.

According to the *British Journal of Pharmacology*, phytocannabinoids is defined as "any plant-derived natural product capable of either directly interacting with cannabinoid receptors or sharing chemical similarity with cannabinoids or both." This includes plants like cloves, rosemary, and hops due to their beta-caryophyllene content—an essential oil that gives these plants their spicy, peppery flavor that has promise as an anti-inflammatory, neuroprotectant, and antidepressant.

Other plants contain- *By giving your dog phy-*
ing cannabinoids in- *tocannabinoids such as*
clude kava, liverwort, *those derived from the can-*
black truffles, and a *nabis plant, your dog can*
variety of sunflower *be a happy, well-balanced*
called *Echinacea Pur-* *pooch.*
pura.

The bodies of dogs actually produce cannabinoids for optimum health and well-being. Because endocannnabinoids like anandamide serve
the important function of regulating pain, hunger,
sleep, and mood, deficiencies in endocannabinoid
production and metabolism can wreak havoc on
the body. But by giving your dog phytocannabinoids such as those derived from the cannabis
plant, your dog can be a happy, well-balanced
pooch.

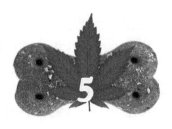

Cannabinoids

Cannabinoid receptors are the most abundant neurotransmitter receptors in the body. When activated, they scan their environment then send the appropriate signals to the appropriate receptors. But just how do different cannabinoids interact with and exert different effects on the body?

The answer to that may be different based on numerous factors such as the individual dog's sensitivity to cannabinoids, the layout of cannabinoid receptors in the body, which varies from dog to dog in much the same way fingerprints do, and which cannabinoids are at play.

Endogenous Cannabinoids

We humans and our dogs create endogenous cannabinoids in our bodies to maintain homeostasis. Individual cannabinoids exert different outcomes by activating different cannabinoid receptors throughout the body. For example, the activation of CB1 Receptors in the brain and spinal cord regulate the uptake of neurotransmitters like serotonin and dopamine while CB2 receptor activation results in more localized, anti-inflammatory responses.

Cannabinoid Receptors

- CB1 receptor activation in the brain and spinal cord regulate the uptake of neurotransmitters like serotonin and dopamine.

- CB2 receptor activation results in more localized, anti-inflammatory responses.

A review from Masaryk University explains, "The activation of cannabinoid CB1 receptors results in retrograde inhibition of the neuronal release of acetylcholine, dopamine, GABA, histamine, serotonin, glutamate, cholecystokinin, D-aspartate, glycine and noradrenaline ... CB2 receptors localized mainly in cells associated with the immune

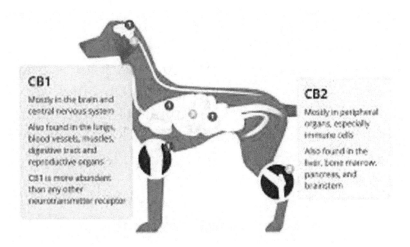

CB1

Mostly in the brain and central nervous system

Also found in the lungs, blood vessels, muscles, digestive tract and reproductive organs

CB1 is more abundant than any other neurotransmitter receptor

CB2

Mostly in peripheral organs, especially immune cells

Also found in the liver, bone marrow, pancreas, and brainstem system are involved in the control of inflammatory processes."

This explains the importance of cannabinoids and highlights the potential of cannabis therapy, but it should be noted that cannabinoid supplementation is just that: supplementing phyto- or synthetic cannabinoids for the real thing. In healthy individuals—both humans and dogs, the endogenous production of cannabinoids is typically sufficient.

The specific cannabinoids produced by the body seem to be consistent throughout many species, though more research is needed to understand variations and how they relate to trends among the species. For example, humans and dogs both experience an increase in endocannabinoid production after rigorous exercise resulting in "runner's high" whereas other animals like ferrets do not.

Anthropologist David A. Raichlen found that endocannabinoid levels in the blood were significantly increased for both humans and dogs—both of which are animals with limbs that have evolved for running—after 30 minutes on a treadmill, while ferrets—animals that have not evolved such traits—did not. Researchers suggest the increased endocannabinoid production may have evolved as a way to "reward" or encourage physical activity in cursorial mammal. i.e., to help them save themselves in case they need to run from predators.

What Endocannabinoids Do

Scientists have identified five endogenous cannabinoids to date—plus a number of fatty acids that help metabolize said cannabinoids, the most prominent of those being anandamide (AEA) and 2-Arachidonoylglycerol (2-AG). Though research is limited regarding their specific role, our knowledge of them is expanding quickly. Here's what we know so far about the five endogenous cannabinoids that have been studied.

Anandamide (AEA)

The neurotransmitter, anandamide, derived its name from the Sanskrit word for "joy" or "bliss" and has been credited for its ability to reduce anxiety and depression by modulating the uptake of neurotransmitters like dopamine and serotonin. It has been shown to impair working memory in rats—though the evolutionary necessity of this has yet to be understood—and plays a vital role in fertility and fetal development as evident in its spike during ovulation. Though it has been suggested that anandamide could be a biomarker of infertility, the theory has yet to be confirmed scientifically.

Interestingly, anandamide is not exclusive to animal production. Chocolate has also been shown to contain AEA—in addition to two other chemicals that mimic AEA in the body—which may explain why we feel better after a chocolate snack. Truffles, though containing no AEA, have been shown to boost natural anandamide production.

2-Arachidonoylglycerol (2-AG)

2-Arachidonoylglycerol (2-AG) is an endogenous cannabinoid that modulates the functionality of other cannabinoids. Unlike AEA, 2-AG is a full agonist of CB1 receptors in the brain and is the primary ligand, or binding molecule, for CB2 receptors throughout the rest of the body. Concentration levels of 2-AG in the brain are around 170 percent higher than anandamide!

Whereas anandamide is produced by the body "on demand", the production of 2-AD is based on an internal clock, regulating things like appetite, sleep cycle, bone health and so on. 2-AG can be found in high concentrations in both human and bovine (cattle) milk, which likely helps regulate the sleeping/feeding cycle of young infants.

2-Arachidonyl Glyceryl Ether (2-AGE)

Also known as noladin ether, 2-Arachidonyl glyceryl ether (2-AGE) is a lesser-known endocannabinoid that is only present in some animals—like dogs and humans, but not others—like hamsters and guinea pigs. It binds to CB1 receptors to reduce blood pressure and relieve pain. In high doses, it can cause sedation, reduced body temperature, and intestinal immobility.

Virodhamine (O-AEA)

Virodhamine (O-AEA) is a cannabinoid that functions opposite of anandamide – it blocks CB1 receptors and activates CB2 receptors in peripheral tissue. Though it is a secondary CB1 cannabinoid (anandamide being the primary), it's concentration of up to two to nine times that of AEA in peripheral tissue suggests it may be primary cannabinoid for CB2 receptors, responsible for helping regulate body temperature.

N-arachidonoyl Dopamine (NADA)

N-arachidonoyl dopamine (NADA) activates CB receptors throughout the brain and body to facilitate some responses. For example, it acts as a potent anti-inflammatory, neuroprotectant, and antioxidant, and also helps coordinate muscle movement and blood flow. It's activation of the vanilloid 1 (TRPV1) receptor also suggests it plays a role in the mediation of pain and thermosensitivity.

Phytocannabinoids and the Body

More than 120 different cannabinoids have been discovered in the cannabis plant, the first of which—and the whole reason the endocannabinoid system began being studied in the first place—is (−)-trans-Δ^9-tetrahydrocannabinol or THC. Though it's fairly common knowledge that THC causes a "high" when smoked or ingested, other benefits of adding plant-derived cannabinoids are being studied, as well—with interesting results, too! Here are seven of the most common cannabinoids found in cannabis along with some proposed therapeutic applications.

Tetrahydrocannabinolic Acid (THCa)

Tetrahydrocannabinolic Acid, or THCa, is the precursor to THC. In other words, THCa is simply THC before the extra carboxyl atom has been removed, a process that happens naturally over time or it can be expedited just by adding a little heat.

Though THCa is not psychoactive, it shows a lot of therapeutic promise. The fact that it is not yet psychoactive means that it can provide even more therapeutic potential for a higher dose than of THC itself without the unwanted side effects.

Juicing raw cannabis enables a full spectrum of cannabinoids to be ingested as a liquid to ward against things like inflammation, neurodegenerative disorders, and even cancer. Other

Juicing raw cannabis enables a full spectrum of cannabinoids to be injected daily to ward against things like inflammation, neurodegenerative disorders, and even cancer

medical benefits of THCa include pain control, improved sleep, and reduced muscle spasms.

Tetrahydrocannabinol (THC)

With a little heat and time, THCa transforms into THC, causing cetain major physiological changes as a result. Commonly referred to as being "high" or "stoned" the consumption of THC can affect memory, movement, time perception, and anxiety levels while contributing to feelings of euphoria, creativity, or varied levels of alertness. Some people describe the "high" sensation as if they were floating around their world, perceiving their surroundings from a whole new perspective.

The high is not THC's only effect. When consumed in low to moderate doses, THC can help control nausea and promote appetite while improving metabolism, lessen both general and localized pain perception, reduce inflammation, control epilepsy, minimize glaucoma, ease depression and anxiety, help with substance dependency and withdraw, and more! Research also suggests that THC's ability to affect memory may be beneficial in the treatment of PTSD, as well.

Cannabinol (CBN)

As THC degrades, it becomes cannabinol or CBN. CBN is only mildly psychoactive but has major sedative properties, i.e., old weed = sleepy weed.

Old weed = Sleepy weed. It increases appetite
**   *CBN is helpful in*** and reduces inflam-
**   *treating insomnia.*** mation and may be
beneficial in the treatment of asthma by reducing
mucus build-up in the lungs.

Though people often imagine old, stale cannabis when thinking of CBN, more growers are selecting it for high CBN strains to offer the benefits
of the chemical without the sometimes overpow-
ering high that accompanies it. CBN is especially
helpful in the treatment of insomnia.

Cannabidiolic Acid (CBDa)

THCa is to THC what Cannaidiolic Acid (CBDa)
is to CBD. It is the precursor to CBD, and its extra
atom is its major distinguishing factor. Though
there are some medical benefits to the consumption of CBDa, we don't know much about the
extent of those properties. For example, though
CBDa has anti-cancer and anti-inflammatory
properties, little else has been scientifically prov-
en. However, some researchers suggest that CBDa
has painkilling, anti-nausea, antioxidant, and
antibacterial features, as well.

Cannabidiol (CBD)

Cannabidiol, or CBD, is the second most popular
cannabinoid next to THC. CBD has been shown to
have incredible medicinal potential by mediating

intracellular communication. Because it is not psy-choactive, CBD can provide the therapeutic poten-tial to a wide range of patients including children, the elderly, and, yes, even your precious pooch. In fact, because CBD acts as an antagonist of CB re-ceptors—it blocks them thereby controlling what activates cannabinoid receptors and what doesn't. CBD helps to reduce unwanted side effects of THC.

Research has shown CBD to hold promise in the treatment of pain, anxiety, depression, inflam-mation, fungal and bacterial infections, neuro-logical disorders, bone regeneration, cancer cell apoptosis, the prevention diabetic disorders, and dementia caused by brain injury or swelling. CBD has also been shown to help regenerate brain cells to help improve recovery after injury or hypemic hypoxia—oxygen loss—in the brain.

Cannabigerol (CBG)

Cannabis is only one source of *Cannabigerol* (CBG); the Southern Africa flower, Helichrysum umbraculigerum, also contains CBG. But, no matter its source, CBG holds great promise for medicinal applications. Thought to be a precursor to cannabinoids like THCa and CBDa, CBG helps alleviate neuropathic pain, especially in areas where other cannabinoids like CBD lack. It may also help control digestion problems by reducing swelling along the gastrointestinal tract.

Cannabichromene (CBC)

Cannabichromene (CBC) is another important phytocannabinoid from the cannabis plant but unlike other cannabinoids, it does not interact directly with cannabinoid receptors. Instead, CBC interacts with receptors like TRPV1 and TRPA1 to help increase the body's own endocannabinoid levels by interfering with the enzymes that break them down.

CBC can be used to stimulate bone growth, prevent or treat diarrhea, reduce swelling, stave off bacterial and fungal infections, treat depression and anxiety, minimize pain perception, and kill cancer cells.

Customized Cannabinoid Profiles

Technology has come a long way, allowing cannabis manufactures to isolate specific cannabinoids and terpenes directly from the cannabis plant, which helps consumers customize their cannabinoid consumption, but breeders have been doing this, too, by selecting cannabis strains with the best features to carry on their lineage.

Breeders cross the best strains with other strains until developing the perfect combination of cannabinoids, terpenes and, in some cases, aesthetics, as well. Though the phenotype varies by plant, many of a strains best features are passed down through the generations to give you the option to choose the best strains —and thus the best cannabinoid profile—for your dog's particular needs.

For those planning on using cannabis flower to treat your dog's discomfort—especially if you'll be growing your own—pay special attention to the strains typical cannabinoid content rather than just a fancy name or pretty photo. Leafly on line has strain reviews, which are helpful in zeroing in on strains with special qualities.

Warning: Synthetic Cannabinoids

There are hundreds of synthetic cannabinoids on the market with new ones being introduced regularly. These man-made chemicals are considered cannabinoids because of their ability to interact with cannabinoid receptors, but they are not all created equal.

Importantly, synthetic cannabinoids should be approved by a vet because some are not fit for consumption.

Unlike other cannabinoids, synthetic cannabinoids bind fully to cannabinoid receptors and can cause a wide variety of reactions—many of which may not be safe. If you are planning on giving your dog synthetic cannabinoids, be sure they come from a reliable source and have ample research to back them. Marinol (dronabinol) and Cesamet (nabilone) are the only FDA approved synthetic cannabinoids and have not been tested on dogs. It is probably wise to avoid synthetic cannabinoids with dogs until more research is available.

Risks of Cannabis

Size matters! Importantly, size plays a significant role in how cannabis effects dogs. If your dog is small, you could easily weight as much as ten times that of your dog—or more. Dog owners need to be cautious when administering cannabis edibles to their pooches because a single cookie potent enough to get a 150-pound human "stoned" could have 10 times that effect on a 15-pound dog.

The smaller the dog, the greater the effect that a small edible will have on it. If two dogs—one 10 years old, 80 pounds and the other 6 weeks old, 5 pounds—get into the same size stash, the smaller dog will have a different reaction compared to that of the larger dog.

How Cannabis Effects Dogs

The ingestion of too much cannabis can be life threatening to your dog. Although cannabis has a large safety margin, it can still make your dog

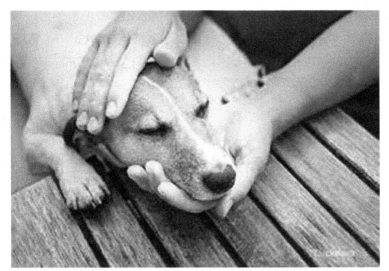

Always start low and go slow.

quite ill and neurologically impaired. Some dogs become anxious and afraid after getting high, which is exhibited by panting and pacing. We can't determine which dogs will become "paranoid" until they are high. Baked laced goods present the most danger because a dog will eat the entire supply, if able, which may be well over an "overdose". which is especially toxic if it includes chocolate.

The A.S.P.C.A. poison center reports that dogs account for about 95 percent of pet cannabis poisonings. The Medical Director, Tina Wismer, of the A.S.P.C.A.'s national animal poison center said she did not know of a death from a dog eating cannabis that did not involve chocolate, which is highly toxic to dogs. Ed-

Ingestion of too much cannabis can be life threatening to your dog.

ibles high in THC concentrations are the most
dangerous to dogs, especially when combined
with brownies, chocolate, or raisin cookies. The
reaction could range from sickening to dying.

Symptoms of THC Overdose

- Severe depression
- Walking drunk—loss of balance
- Lethargy
- Coma
- Low heart rate
- Low blood pressure
- Dilated pupils
- Coma
- Hyperactivity
- Vocalization
- Seizures
- Breathing problems
- Abnormal heart rhythms
- Urinary incontinence

When ingestion of cannabis was recent, treatment
usually involves inducing vomiting, then keeping
the dog in a quiet place and hydrated until the
cannabis passes through the it's system, which can
take a couple of days in some cases.

Dogs Do Not React Like Humans

Realistically, it is unlikely that your dog will die—fortunately! For marijuana intake to be lethal, your furry friend would have to be a small-sized dog, ingesting at least one pound or more of high THC edibles or buds. At this level, danger is real.

A study published in the *Journal of Veterinary Emergency and Critical Care* in 2012 analyzed experiences of 125 dogs in Colorado that had ingested cannabis between 2005 and 2010. The researchers

There is no way to anticipate how your dog will respond to a cannabis overdose.

concluded that ingesting baked goods made with tetrahydrocannabinol butter lead to the death of 2 dogs. However, the report concluded that the dogs died from asphyxiating on their own vomit. One dog asphyxiated after ingesting an entire pound of pot brownies, whereas the other dog had ingested a pound of pot butter.

In 2013 researchers Fitzgerald, Bronstein and Newquist reported in *Top Companion Animal Medicine,* "The minimum lethal oral dose for dogs for THC is more than 3 g/kg. Although the cannabis has a high margin of safety, deaths have been seen after ingestion of food products containing the more concentrated medical-grade THC butter."

This is quite a different story from a 1973 submission, in which scientists wrote in the *Journal*

Toxicology and Applied Pharmacology that "In dogs and monkeys, single oral doses of Δ^9-THC and Δ^8-THC between 3000 and 9000 mg/kg were non-lethal." Fitzgerald concludes that while second-hand smoke inhalation is possible, the most common source of exposure to cannabis is through ingestion of the dog owner's supply.

In short, 44 years ago, ingesting 3 to 9 grams of THC per kilogram of your dog's body weight would not kill it, but in 2013, 3 grams of THC per kg of your dog's body weight is considered the minimum lethal dose. This discrepancy may be partially explained by the increasing potency of THC in cannabis in recent years as compared to back in the 1970s. While evidence is suggesting that dogs have a lower tolerance than do humans for THC, the psychoactive ingredient in pot, because of the paucity of research, scientists just don't know the lethal doses for dogs of various sizes.

There is no way to anticipate how your dog will respond to a cannabis overdose, especially considering the size of your dog and what else it may have ingested with the pot. If you suspect your pup has gotten into your stash, especially if it has ingested chocolate along with the weed, take it to your vet, ASAP.

How to Treat Overdose

Take your dog to the vet immediately. Vets will usually try to induce vomiting in your dog to get whatever it's eaten out of its system. If your dog is lethargic—a sign that the THC is already in its bloodstream—do not try to induce vomiting because the dog could swallow its vomit and asphyxiate. After clearing the stomach, vets then watch for seizures, which can happen if they ate *a lot* of weed and give them fluids to clear its system faster. After that you must watch and wait because there is no antidote to reverse the effects of marijuana.

No matter what illegal substances your dog may have ingested take your dog to a vet and tell the vet exactly what it might have in its system—even if it is something *You must watch and wait because there is no antidote to reverse the effects of THC.* illegal that you should not have let them get into. Your dog can't be treated if the vet doesn't have *all* the information.

Can Cannabis Kill My Dog?

It takes *a lot* of weed to kill a dog. We do know that extremely an high level of THC in cannabis is toxic to dogs, but research has yet to determine whether or not THC is the primary cause of death, or whether ingesting other toxins along with the marijuana, such as chocolate, is more to blame. In any case owners should be vigilant, especially if you have a small, old or sick dog.

While there is a general view that cannabis is fully safe, it isn't.

—Dr. Gary Richter

"A Colorado study showed a four-fold increase in cannabis-related overdose cases, and much of that is ascribed to pets getting into their owners' stash", according to Ken Pawlowski, past president of the California Veterinary Medical Association. Dogs appear to be even more susceptible because they have more cannabinoid receptors, Pawlowski said. He is concerned about the lack of oversight in the proliferation of cannabis in canine products.

President of the California Veterinary Medical Association, Kevin D. Lazarcheff reported seeing intoxications associated with the purposeful use of 'low THC' cannabinoid or CBD products." Onset of symptoms after ingesting or inhaling marijuana is 30 to 60 minutes in most dogs. Depending on the dosage and strength of the weed, signs can last from 18 to 36 hours.

Dr. Gary Richter a 20-year veterinarian and Medical Director of Montclair Veterinary Hospital and of the Holistic Veterinary Care of Oakland believes there is an enormous potential to treat medical conditions in canines with cannabis. Richter warns that while there is a general view that cannabis is fully safe, it isn't. He says THC can be dangerous to dogs, leading to medical complications and, in extreme cases, even to death. An overdose can cause loss of balance and possible collapse, even death in rare cases.

Avoid Chocolate

Theobromine in chocolate is poisonous to dogs. However, the degree of hazard to your dog depends on the type of chocolate, the amount consumed and your dog's size. In large enough amounts, chocolate and cocoa products can kill your dog. Both caffine and theobromine are used medicinally as a diuretic, heart stimulant, blood vessel dilator, and a smooth muscle relaxant. Dogs cannot metabolize theobromine and caffeine as well as people do. This makes them more sensitive to the chemicals' effects.

Why Not Chocolate?

• Humans easily metabolize theobromine, but dogs process it much more slowly, allowing it to build up to toxic levels in their system.

• A large dog can consume more chocolate than a small dog before suffering ill effects.

• A small amount of chocolate will probably only give your dog an upset stomach with vomiting or diarrhea.

- In large amounts, theobromine can produce muscle tremors, seizures, an irregular heartbeat, internal bleeding or a heart attack.

- The onset of theobromine poisoning is usually marked by severe hyperactivity.

- If you have a small dog that has eaten a box of chocolates, you need to go to your veterinarian right away. Do not wait.

The amount and type of chocolate ingested is also important, as they are the determining factors for the severity of the toxicity.

Milk Chocolate

Mild signs of toxicity can occur when 0.7 ounces per pound of body weight is ingested; severe toxicity occurs when two ounces per pound of body weight is ingested—or as little as one pound of milk chocolate for a 20-pound dog.

Semi-Sweet Chocolate

Mild signs of toxicity can occur when 0.3 ounce per pound of body weight is ingested; severe toxicity occurs when one ounce per pound of body weight is ingested—or as little as six ounces of semi-sweet chocolate for a 20-pound dog.

Baking Chocolate

This type of chocolate has the highest concentration of caffeine and theobromine. Therefore, as little as two small one-ounce squares of baking chocolate can be toxic to a 20-pound dog—or 0.1 ounce per pound of body weight.

Important: If you suspect that your dog may have eaten a large quantity of chocolate and is showing any of the signs listed below, call your veterinarian immediately.

The usual treatment for theobromine poisoning is to induce vomiting within two hours of ingestion.

Different chocolate types have different theobromine levels. Cocoa, cooking chocolate and dark chocolate contain the highest levels of theobromine, while milk chocolate and white chocolate have the lowest.

Always err on the side of caution when dealing with any quantity of dark or bitter chocolate. The high level of theobromine in dark chocolate means it takes only a very small amount to poison a dog. Less than an ounce of dark chocolate may be enough to poison a 44-pound dog.

Symptoms of Chocolate Poisoning

- Vomiting
- Diarrhea
- Increased body temperature
- Increased reflex responses
- Muscle rigidity
- Rapid breathing
- Increased heart rate
- Low blood pressure
- Seizures
- Cardiac failure
- Weakness
- Coma

Never consider chocolate as a reward. Instead give your dog healthy treats along with lots of love and attention.

Other Foods to Avoid

- **Alcohol** can cause vomiting, diarrhea, decreased coordination, central nervous system depression, difficulty breathing, tremors, abnormal blood acidity, coma and even death

- **Coffee & Caffine** products all contain substances called methylxanthines. When injested it can cause vomiting and diarrhea, panting, excessive thirst and urination, hyperactivity, abnormal heart rhythm, tremors, seizures and even death

• **Coconut oil.** The flesh and milk of fresh coconuts do contain oils that may cause stomach upset, loose stools or diarrhea. Coconut water is high in potassium and should not be given to your dog.

• **Milk and Dairy.** Because dogs do not possess significant amounts of lactase—the enzyme that breaks down lactose in milk, milk and other dairy-based products cause them diarrhea or other digestive upset.

• **Onions, Garlic Chives** can cause gastro-intestinal irritation and could lead to red blood cell damage

• **Raw-Uncooked Meat, Eggs and Bones** can contain bacteria such as Salmonella and E. coli that can be harmful to pets and humans. salt & salty snack food

• **Xylitol** is a sweetener found in many products, including gum, candy, baked goods and toothpaste. It can cause insulin release in most species, which can lead to liver failure. The increase in insulin leads to hypoglycemia—lowered sugar levels. Initial signs of toxicosis include vomiting, lethargy and loss of coordination. Can progress to seizures

• **Yeast Dough** can rise and cause gas to accumulate in your dog's digestive system. This can be painful and can cause the stomach to bloat, and potentially twist, becoming a life threatening emergency

Be Safe; Not Sorry

Keep these out of reach of your dog. Be especially careful to clear off the dining table when moving to the living room. You know how dogs are. Leave some cookies on the table to to TV chair when going to bed, and your pooch will likely climb into your chair and scarf them down. Keep you dog healthy and happy!

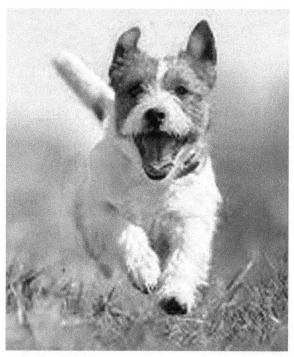

Keep your dog happy and healthy.

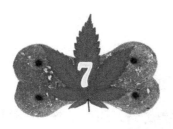

Cannabis & the Law

In the 1936's the scare movie, *Reefer Madness* swept the states as newspapers reported the "dangers of marijuana." Specifically, anti-pot propaganda purported that marijuana would make users lazy and crazy, and ultimately invite in the Devil. *Reefer Madness* depicted innocent children being lured into buying "marihuana", which was a slang term for cannabis in Mexico. Smoking the weed turned one into a violent, psychotic, sex-driven lunatic. The movie showed users committing horrific acts of violence including manslaughter, suicide, and attempt-

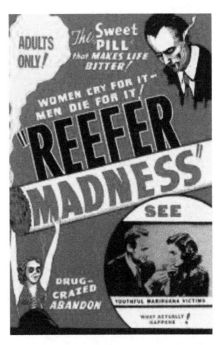

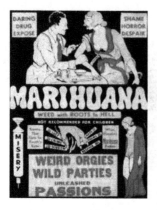

ed rape, and suggested that the hallucinations induced by marijuana were enough to drive one crazy.

Such "yellow journalism" was effective and continued for decades backed in large part by Harry J. Anslinger, the first Commissioner of the Federal Bureau of Narcotics. Anslinger was a key player in the production and promotion of *Reefer Madness* as well as many other anti-pot films like *Assassin of Youth* and *Marihuana* which effectively scared the public—and politicians—into a near century-long fear of cannabis use.

Cannabis Criminalized

Concerns regarding research that linked marijuana to crime and other socially deviant behavior led to the passing of the *Marijuana Tax Act in 1937*, which criminalizied use of cannabis for anyone who wasn't medically registered to use it. Hemp, however, was still legal and still encouraged to grow. Both marijuana and hemp come from the same genus—cannabis. Before the *Reefer Madness* scare marijuana was called cannabis and found in many doctor's medical bag to be used as a reliable palliative. Interestingly, in recent years marijuana is increasingly called "cannabis".

While marijuana can have high levels of THCa, whereas hemp contains less than .3 percent THCa. Hemp is loaded with CBD and other cannainoids, making hemp-based cannabis products safe for dogs.

Hemp is an excellent source of fiber and new technology makes it easier to process. World War II marked the last push for local hemp production with the federal government encouraging cultivation of hemp—as long as they promised not to use it as an intoxicant, along with production of hemp processing factories. Unfortunately, the war ended before many of these facilities were completed leaving farmers high and dry with half-built factories and canceled hemp contracts.

During the 1950's marijuana use continued despite growing public disapproval, so Congress introduced stricter sentencing laws to help reduce its appeal. Some of the mandatory sentencing for drug convictions, which covered marijuana, included prison time and fines of up to $20,000—a lot of money in the 1950s—for first-time possession charges.

Despite all this, marijuana use grew in popularity. In the 1960's and 70's, many pop culture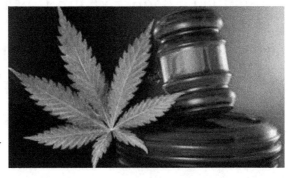

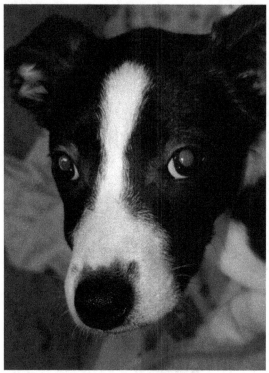

Disney as a pup.

figures like Timothy Leary with his slogan: "Tune On, Turn In, Drop Out" and anti-war groups actively promoted the use of marijuana and faced legal action for doing so, including raids, prison time and deportation.

Marijuana use continued to soar, prompting many researchers to readdress past studies claiming its detriment. Things were going great. Marijuana was showing promise with minimal risks and people loved it.

But then it happened. In 1970, President Richard Nixon signed into law *The Controlled Substance Act* which listed cannabis—specifically due to THC's psychoactive properties—as a Schedule I narcotic defined as *a substance with the most potential for abuse, with no medical value* right alongside LSD, heroin, and cocaine.

By listing cannabis as a Schedule I drug, researchers were forced to jump through numerous hoops to get the approval, funding, and materials needed to scientifically study the plant's chemical composition and effects on the body. So research into cannabis' beneficial qualities dried up—especially as it relates to our beloved dogs. Vets can actually lose their license if they prescribe cannabis.

Schedule I Narcotic

The Controlled Substance Act is intended to make it easier to track, regulate, and enforce drugs and their corresponding policies. This federal drug policy was designed to help regulate the production and distribution of controlled substances by categorizing them into one of five "schedules." Schedule I, for example, contains drugs that have no accepted medical value, a high potential for abuse, and pose a significant risk to one's safety. Schedule II drugs have a high potential for abuse and potential for dependence, Schedule III a low potential for abuse or dependence, and so on.

The problem is that THC, the main psychoactive chemical in cannabis, has landed marijuana on the list of most dangerous drugs. Thus rendering *all cannabinoids* from the cannabis plant as Schedule I since it is "cannabis" that is listed and not "THC". Marijuana's schedule status not only makes it difficult to acquire cannabis but also makes it extremely difficult to research it. Unfortunately, without adequate research, cannabis may not be able to make it off Schedule I.

Catch 22

Cannabis's Schedule I status puts it into a Catch-22. For there to be proven medical value, there needs to be adequate research. However, to conduct scientifically relevant research, the study must first be approved; cannabis acquired; and sample population size big enough, diverse enough, and be willing to participate long enough to extrapolate the appropriate data. Even if able to get past the first two hurdles—which are both lengthy and difficult, the third—keeping study participants actually participating—is still a major challenge given the legal status of cannabis. Fear of legal or social repercussions limits both the diversity of participants and their long-term commitment to the study.

Though some suggest rescheduling cannabis to a Schedule II drug to make research easier, others are concerned that doing so could put a monopoly on the budding industry by blocking entrepreneurs because Schedule II drugs require lengthy, costly research and regulations to be distributed to a large population. The alternative would be to deschedule marijuana—remove it from the list of schedules altogether—and to opt instead for state-mandated cannabis laws as is the case with liquor and tobacco.

Legal Status & Research

More research is needed. Yet, from a historical perspective, cannabis is one of the most widely researched drugs out there. Cannabis use has been documented for centuries and may well be one of the most diverse forms of therapy known to man. But until it's legal status is lifted, it will be difficult to acquire the information needed to understand the complexities of this amazing plant.

Fortunately, with cannabis legalization sweeping the nation, many of the current barriers researchers have faced are being lifted. People can self-medicate without fear of government intervention, and researchers can legally acquire the funding—and product needed to test large populations.

However, research regarding our canine companions is likely to be a few years off, hence the appeal of conducting our own—alongside veterinary guidance, of course. Though your vet may not be able to *recommend* cannabis therapy for your dog, he or she should be able to help you monitor treatment options and adjust your methods accordingly.

Though the future of cannabis is promising, its legal status has slowed our understanding of the plant hence the importance of careful, home-based cannabis experiments.

Ending Federal Marijuana Prohibition

Representatives Tom Garrett (R-VA) and Tulsi Gabbard (D-HI) have introduced comprehensive marijuana reform legislation, the *Ending Federal Marijuana Prohibition Act of 2017, HR 1227*. This Act eliminates federal criminal penalties for possessing and growing marijuana. This legislation gives states the power and flexibility to establish their own marijuana policies free from federal interference. The bill would also remove marijuana from the *Controlled Substances Act*, which would allow for more marijuana research both recreationally and medicinally.

Surprising many, Senate Minority leader Chuck Schumer (D-NY) has publicly announced his intent to sponsor legislation to remove marijuana from the federal *Controlled Substances Act.*

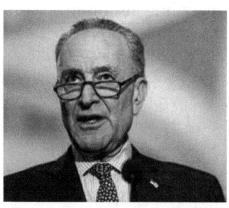

Schumer has communicated that it is a legislative priority for the Democratic Party to end the federal prohibition of marijuana. All of which suggests there will be changes in laws regarding marijuana in the coming years—hopefully.

Senator Schumer supports removing marijuana from federal regulation.

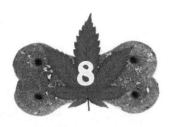

Work with Your Vet

After decades of anti-pot propaganda, it's no wonder the evolution of the cannabis movement has been slow going. Not only has cannabis prohibition essentially frozen research, but it has struck fear into the hearts of thousands across the globe regarding the safety of cannabis consumption.

While advocacy has made great strides in the right to consume cannabis for medicinal purposes with humans, such is not the case for our canine friends. Our dogs do not have a right to consume cannabis or cannabis extracts. Of course, this doesn't deter the private distribution of cannabis to canines, it does prevent veterinarians from prescribing, recommending, or even discussing cannabis therapy with patients and their owners. Because cannabis is classified as a Schedule 1 narcotic, which restricts use even by researchers, veterinarians and researchers can't determine the level of toxicity or doses.

Medical Use Not Legal for Dogs

In 1996, California became the first US state to legalize the medical use of cannabis. Since then, more than half of States have legalized cannabis in some capacity, most frequently for medical purposes. But in all the efforts to push for the right of humans to use medical marijuana, activists neglected to include dogs, our best friends, in the legal framework.

Despite an abundance of pot products for dogs, the FDA does not approve cannabis for animals, which translates to an abundance of pet pot products without regulatory over-site: Outlaw products. Products may contain inconsistent cannabinoid concentrations or inconsistent dosing instructions, for example, or they may contain additives not recommended for dog consumption—especially if they've been imported from overseas.

Furthermore, because there is little research and therefore little known about proper canine dosing, products marketed to dog owners may suggest using quantities that are either unsafe or ineffective. This is important to note given dogs' increased sensitivity to cannabinoids because of having a larger concen-

The FDA does not approve cannabis for animals, which translates to an abundance of pet pot products that have no regulatory oversite: Outlaw Products!

tration of cannabinoid receptors. On top of that a high concentration of cannabinoids—especially THC and its precursor THCa—can be fatal by causing extreme lethargy, confusion, and an increased or sporadic heart rate.

Vets and the Law

Though there is growing support for medicinal cannabis and an increasing anecdotal evidence of its effectiveness in treating canine health problems, the veterinary community is professionally prohibited from discussing it with dog owners. When a client inquires about cannabis therapy for *The veterinary community is professionally prohibited from discussing cannabis with dog owners.* their dog, all a vet is legally allowed to say about it is "I cannot recommend cannabis." Not that they don't recommend it—just that *they literally cannot say anything about cannabis for fear of legal repercussions*, i.e., losing their license.

Even where the State has deemed cannabis use legal for things like glaucoma, cancer pain, and arthritis, veterinarians are barred from having the simple discussion with their clients because of the Schedule I status.

Because cannabis is classified as a Schedule I narcotic on par with heroin and LSD, which implies it has "no medical value," obtaining the funding needed to conduct scientifically valid

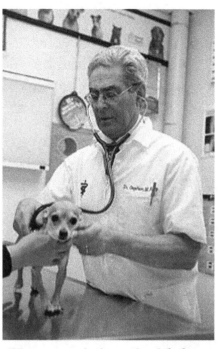

Vet examining timid dog.

research is both difficult and time-consuming. As a result little research has been done on canines. Little is known about the makeup of the canine endocannabinoid system or how dogs differ from humans and other animal models. This makes establishing standardized dosing and toxicity levels difficult, putting veterinarians at great risk should they misdose.

Under the guidance of the American Veterinarian Medical Board, practitioners can be punished for misconduct by revoking a license, suspending it indefinitely, or other disciplinary action based on state-specific laws. Considering what a veterinarian spends in student loans on their 5 to 9-year degree program, it's no wonder so many are reluctant to discuss medicinal cannabis with their canine caregivers.

More Rights for Vets

As medical marijuana legislation spreads across the nation, it's only natural for people to want to share their new-found freedom with their canines, which is not surprising considering the abundance of cannabis products marketed exclusively to dogs.

The number of cannabis products for dogs has significantly grown since legalization took hold, and with seemingly great results. Anecdotal evidence suggests that cannabis extracts help dogs live longer, happier, healthier lives by adding a few cannabinoids to their daily diet.

But product manufacturers and distributors are not medical professionals. They do not have the intimate knowledge that veterinarians have regarding what is and isn't safe, normal, or concerning regarding our dogs and certainly don't have the dedication to your dog's well-being that veterinarians have, either. In fact, there may be no greater animal advocate than a veterinarian who has dedicated his or her life to helping animals. To stifle their ability to openly discuss an herb that is already being used by thousands of people is both destructive and unfair to our furry friends who look to us to protect their well-being.

Many vets across the nation are speaking out about the discrepancy regarding medical marijuana for dogs. According to Liz Hughston, founder of VetTechXpert and administrator of the social media group, Veterinary Cannabis Academy, "I think we've reached an inflection point in society now where cannabis use in humans has become much more widespread and accepted. People see the good it does in people and want to provide the same benefits to their pets."

But cannabis does not have the same effect on dogs as it does humans, and it's important for veterinarians to explain this to their canine caregivers. High doses of THC, for example, can cause extreme disorientation, loss of balance and lethargy. In some cases, high doses of THC in dogs may be fatal if the dog vomits and is too incapacitated to remove itself so chokes.

Though many cannabis products that do not contain THC and are still effective, the lack of

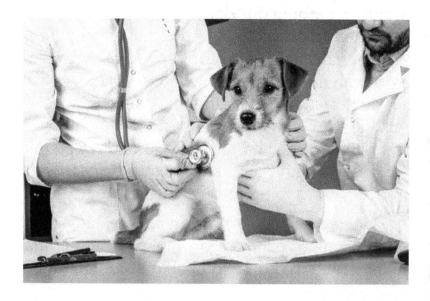

research and regulatory over-site for these canine cannabis products renders our dogs vulnerable to mislabeling and improper dosing. Until veterinarians can provide over-site for cannabis therapy, people will continue to roll the dice in hopes of improving their dog's health. In the meantime, veterinarians across the board recommend using only hemp-based cannabis products that contain an abundance of CBD with little to no THC. The hemp offers many of the same therapeutic benefits as THC—anti-anxiety, pain relief, or increased appetite for example—but do not cause a "high."

"We lack the science to support [the] use of medical marijuana products like CBD oils, not because researchers are unwilling to do the work, but because of bureaucratic red tape and over-regulation."

—Orrin Hatch
Utah Senator

States Rights for Dogs

As of this writing, Colorado is the only state to allow veterinarians to discuss cannabis with their patients. This means that dogs in states like California, Washington, and Maine risk misinformation from marketers rather than medical professionals, but that's not stopping advocates in these States from seeking change.

In early 2018, California Assemblymember, Ash Kalra proposed bill AB-2215 that will allow licensed veterinarians to "discuss the use of cannabis on animal patient clients and…protect state-licensed veterinarians from disciplinary action for discussing the use of cannabis on animal patient clients."

While AB-2215 is backed by California's Veterinary Medical Board, it is considered controversial. Specifically, the majority of Board Members believe the wording is too vague, which could result in substandard safety practices for veterinary professionals. Some vets argue that simply "discussing" cannabis is not sufficient regulatory framework to be effective. The Board insists on maintaining the authority to discipline licensed veterinary practitioners in the event of unsafe dosing recommendations.

Opening up the discussion is an important first step, however. Until the research catches up, many veterinarians simply cannot take the risk of misdosing a dog. Simply discussing cannabis is neither a prescription nor a recommendation, but can still include dosing suggestions, application methods, and cautionary tips to help ensure our dogs remain safe and healthy.

California isn't the only state pushing for change. Researchers studying the effects of cannabidiol on canines were forced to cease research in 2017 when the DEA declared that all cannabinoids, not just THC, are federally-illegal. This has forced many researchers to halt their work while they re-await government approval. The blessing in disguise is that the DEA crackdown inspired dozens of lawmakers across the nation to propose legislation that would make it easier to study the effects of various cannabinoids on dogs.

According to Utah Senator, Orrin Hatch, "We lack the science to support [the] use of medical marijuana products like CBD oils, not because researchers are unwilling to do the work, but because of bureaucratic red tape and over-regulation." This issue needs to be rectified if we are to protect our furry friends from civilian errors. Until research catches up to demand, people will continue to medicate their dogs with potentially unauthorized or unregulated cannabis products without the guidance of their vets, and vets will remain helpless to do anything about it.

Vets Who Risk It All

Legislators and activists are fighting hard for our right to choose cannabis therapy for our dogs, but they're not the only ones. Some veterinarians are risking their professional license by taking to the front lines for cannabis reform.

One such person, Dr. Jamie Payton of the University of California's Davis Veterinary Medical Teaching Hospital, has taken it upon herself to acquire the study information she needs to make educated conclusions about cannabis therapy for canines.

Davis is in the midst of a first-of-its-kind survey to collect data from people who treat their dogs with cannabis. The survey has currently received more than 1300 respondents who give their sick, suffering dogs cannabis products to ease their discomfort.

Davis is concerned about the number of people she sees self-medicating their dogs with cannabis. As the theory goes, cannabis is medically beneficial to humans so why wouldn't it be beneficial to dogs? But many people don't realize just how powerful some cannabinoids can be for dogs—specifically THC—and may over-dose their small pets in unsafe amounts.

Because dogs cannot voice their discomfort, it is up to the veterinary community to protect our furry companions from mistakes and misinformation, and they cannot do so without the proper research and freedom to prescribe what is needed. The survey is a good first step to acquiring research on the matter and can be conducted without having to wade through miles of red tape to get there.

Another such crusader, Dr. Douglas Kramer, left his veterinary practice to start a mobile holistic veterinary practice in California. After witnessing the amazing results cannabis provided to his terminally-ill Siberian Husky, Kramer felt it important to afford the same opportunities for other California canines to use cannabis. He therefore made it his mission to educate people on the benefits and risks of cannabis for canines, and openly discussed his personal experience with the herb. Kramer conducted a survey on trends regarding cannabis use for dogs and other pets.

According to Kramer,

> "I refuse to condemn my patients to a miserable existence for self-preservation or concerns about what may or may not happen to me as a consequence of my actions. My freedom of speech is clearly protected by the First Amendment to the Constitution. This is an issue of animal welfare, plain and simple. Remaining silent would represent a clear violation of the veterinarian's oath I took when I was admitted into this profession."

Though Kramer faced an untimely death in 2013 at the age of 36, his legacy lives on as one of the first pioneers for medical marijuana and dogs. Though few are bold enough to put their careers on the line as Kramer did, many veterinarians are tired of waiting for Congress to give approval and are taking matters into their own hands.

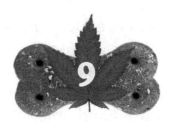

Marijuana or Hemp?

Cannabinoids come from a variety of sources: flowering plants like the Helichrysum flower, fungi like black truffles, and even our own bodies! But the most prominent source of cannabinoids—and the most controversial—are those derived from hemp and from marijuana. But are hemp- and marijuana-based cannabinoids the same thing? Are they both as medicinally relevant? Which can you use safely—and legally— with your best friend?

Hemp

Hemp and marijuana come from the same genus, *Cannabis Sativa L.*—although marijuana also comes from another member of the *Cannabis* family, *Cannabis indica*).

Differences between hemp and marijuana are rooted in their chemical makeup, cultivation practices, and nature of the plant itself. A major difference is that marijuana is the mind-altering

form of can-
nabis, where-
as hemp is a
non-psycho-
active can-
nabis. While
hemp con-
tains many

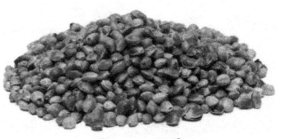

Hemp seeds

cannabinoids, it has little to no THC, the mind-altering cannabinoid.

Hemp is an ideal cash crop because it grows
quickly, replenishes the soil as it grows, and
requires little to no pesticides or fungicides to
thrive. Because hemp is primarily grown for
industrial purposes, it is cultivated in a different way than marijuana. For example, because
marijuana is consumed and used medicinally it
must be cultivated in carefully controlled envi-
ronments. By contrast, hemp plants are typically
densely compacted into large outdoor fields. Hemp

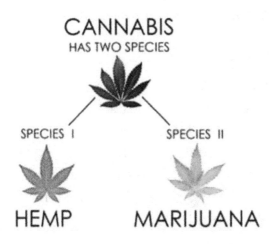

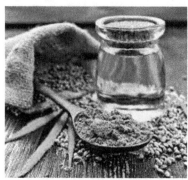

Hemp oil has many therapeutic benefits.

grows tall and slender since the stems and seeds are the most valuable part of the plant. Whereas the flower is a major focus of marijuana, hemp rarely produces flowers.

Only recently has hemp been cultivated for medicinal purposes. For centuries, hemp was grown for its strong fiber, used to create rope, paper, building materials, fabric, paint, plastic, fuel, and more.

Another consideration is that hemp absorbs heavy metals and other contaminants in the soil—which is useful in cleaning up radiation disasters. But when hemp products will be ingested—by humans, especially those intended for medicinal purposes—every step in the process must the thoroughly monitored and carefully cultivated to maintain safety and medical value.

Hemp Oil from Seeds

Hemp seed oil contains the perfect ratio of Omega-6—linoleic acid—to Omega-3—alpha linolenic acid—fatty acids. These are essential fatty acids that your dog must get from its diet to remain in top form. A good balance of these Omega oils is critical to your dog's health because they work synergistically in its body.

Hemp seeds are high in gamma linolenic acid (GLA), which reduces inflammation and strengthens the immune system. Researchers in the *Journal of Arthritis and Rheumatology* found that the GLA in hemp seeds reduced arthritis symptoms and joint pain by 25% in dogs as compared to the placebo at 4%. It also improves skin and coat by reducing the inflammation associated with common · skin issues, including atopic dermatitis, pruritic skin disease and granulomas.

Hemp Legalized

A bipartisan group of U.S. senators introduced *the Industrial Hemp Farming Act of 2014* that allows American farmers to produce and cultivate *industrial* hemp. The bill removes hemp from the Controlled Substances List as long as it contained no more than 0.3 percent THC.

Your dog has substances in its body called "prostaglandins", which are like hormones that circulate around the body, helping to smooth muscle contractions, control inflammation, regulate the body temperature and other vital functions. The GLA that's abundant in hemp seed is a building block for prostaglandins.

Hemp Better for Dogs

Cannabis can have an amazing impact on your dog's health, but not all products are created equal, nor are all cannabinoids. While humans can typically tolerate THC well, dogs cannot. Though research is limited on the subject, the *Canadian Veterinary Journal* suggests dogs have a denser network of cannabinoid receptors that may increase their susceptibility to cannabinoid toxicity.

For this reason, any products containing THC should *not* be given to your dog—including blowing pot smoke in your dog's face. Even if the dog has had THC in the past without complications, the powerful effects of the cannabinoid coupled with your dog's dense network of cannabinoid receptors and an inability to explain the sensations or express discomfort means that THC, though perhaps beneficial for humans, should not be given to your dog. Why risk it?

The contents of any cannabinoid product you will give to your dog must be carefully considered. Edibles are a common method of ingestion and can result in a nasty case of overconsumption and potential food poisoning because dogs will eat all available—the entire plate of brownies, for example. Chocolate is the most common food poison dogs experience, but there are other food products to avoid, including coffee, caffeine, dairy products, onions, garlic, raw or undercooked meat, yeast dough, or excessive amounts of coconut oil.

For all these reasons it makes sense to choose hemp-based products for your dog. Dogs are more sensitive to THC and hemp is low in THC, yet has other beneficial cannabinoids. The most common side effect of CBD is that your dog may get a little drowsy—about the same as if you gave him a Benadryl.

Beware of Fraudlent Products

The Federal Drug Administration has tested many CBD products and has found many to contain less CBD than claimed—some contained no CBD at all!. The FDA has also been reminding many companies that medical claims regarding CBD are prohibited and have issued warning letters to companies infracting upon these standards. However, as CBD's popularity increases—and the scope of the cannabis industry spreads, more and more CBD companies will make their way into the playing field.

Though the FDA works hard to ensure the products on the market are what they say they are, it's always wise to do your due diligence when shopping for CBD-based products for your dog. You can do this by researching CBD companies online, especially their review section and about company page. If the company explains their product in detail, if they tout their testing results, and if they have rave reviews from past customers, you've likely found a solid product. If cultivated and produced locally, all the better.

Availability of Hemp CBD

The vast majority of States have legalized cannabis and cannabis-derived products to some extent for medicinal use only. Some claim that sale of hemp-derived CBD oil is legal in all 50 states as long as it is sold as a dietary supplement in accordance with FDA standards.

CBD is not "legal" in all 50 states—even though it is widely available. The law is murky and open to differing interpretations. Many assert that if the CBD product contains less than 0.3% THC, it is classified as "hemp" under federal law and legal to possess and distribute.

Proponents site the 2014 Farm Bill to support their position that CBD derived from industrial hemp is legal. The legislation, however, legalized only a very narrow set of hemp cultivation activities: Growing hemp under a state pilot program or for academic research and "in which such institution of higher education or state department of agriculture is located and such research occurs."

While there are CBD producers who obtain hemp from cultivators operating under the Farm Bill, it's unlikely that all has been sourced from research hemp. Compounding matters, State laws on hemp-based CBD vary widely. Colorado, which legalized

CBD is not "legal" in all 50 states—even though it is widely available.

adult-use marijuana in 2012, has a strong industrial hemp program, By contrast, in Massachusetts where marijuana can be grown at home, it's still a crime to grow hemp without a State license, according to *The Boston Globe*.

Republican Senator Mitch McConnell has announced that we need a bill to legalize hemp on the federal level. Meanwhile, the Drug Enforcement Administration maintains that CBD is definitely illegal, saying those who violate federal drug law still run the "risk of arrest and prosecution." Although the spokesman, added that the DEA is not going after individuals who have benefited from CBD oil.

"It would not be an appropriate use of federal resources to go after a mother because her child has epileptic seizures and has found something that can help and has helped. Are they breaking the law? Yes, they are. Are we going to break her door down? Absolutely not. And I don't think she'll be charged by any U.S. Attorney," DEA spokesperson Rusty Payne told the Indiana TV News.

Where to Buy Quality CBD

Blake Armstrong, author of the blog, *Cannabis Supplements for Pets*, discovered CBD when his beloved dog, Rosie, was diagnoses with hip dysplasia. He advises to stick with the brands he reviews because they build their products to include ingredients which are beneficial for pets, and their dosage recommendations are specifically for pets.

Armstrong recommends King Kanine's line of CBD oils, balms, sprays, and treats. Infused with top-quality hemp oil, these products are super versatile, easy to use, and reliable. Additonally, all King Kanine products come with dosing information to help you ensure you give your pet the right dose to manage their specific ailment or symptoms.

Armstrong has used with his dog and recommends the products manufactured by Canna-Pet, CBDPet, HolistaPet, Innovet, King Kanine, and Pet Releaf.

Blake Armstrong
recommends:

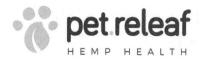 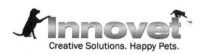

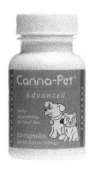 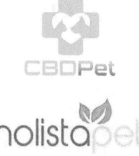 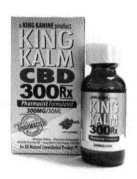

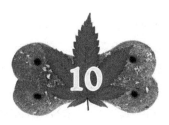

Modes of Administration

For cannabinoids to have their effect, they must find their way into the bloodstream. This can happen in many ways, each method with its own set of benefits and drawbacks. To ensure your pup gets the most benefit from cannabinoid supplementation, be sure to choose the right mode of ingestion.

Inhalation

The best known way to get cannabinoids into the bloodstream is via inhalation. When cannabinoids enter into the lungs by way of smoke or vaporization, they are absorbed into alveoli—tiny air sacks lining the lungs—in a matter of seconds. Due to rapid absorption that the large surface area the alveoli provide, cannabinoids take a few seconds to a few minutes to take effect when

> *For cannabinoids to have their effect, they must find their way into the bloodstream.*

inhaled. Because dogs have greater sensitivity than do humans to cannabinoids—especially the psychoactive cannabinoid, THC—inhalation is not recommended for standard cannabinoid administration. Also, it's not practical since dogs don't smoke.

Typically, dog owners inhale the cannabis themselves then blow it directly into the dog's snout or ear for absorption. Though some dogs don't seem to mind, forcibly restricting a dog to blow an abrasive substance into its lungs could exacerbate anxiety, especially if the smoke or vapor contains high doses of THC.

Experts generally recommend avoiding inhaled cannabis with dogs except under extreme circumstances and only for hemp products that contain little to no THC.

Oral Ingestion

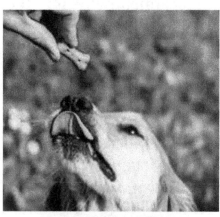

Dogs love edibles.

Cannabis's therapeutic properties are effective when consumed orally, albeit to a different extent. Cannabis that is eaten must be metabolized in the digestive systems before it can be absorbed into the bloodstream, which can take as long as 1 to 2 hours depending on many factors—body weight, metabolic speed, coinciding meals, and lasts for many hours after effects come one. Though this may be ideal for continuous relief, a miscalculated dose or an uncomfortable level of THC could upset little Fido for an extended period of time.

Sublingual Ingestion

Alternatively, cannabinoids may be absorbed sublingually through the mucus membranes inside of the mouth under the tongue. When consumed sublingually, cannabinoids are absorbed directly into the bloodstream quickly, generally around 10 to 15 minutes.

Sublingual cannabis products have a greater bioavailability, which means that less is needed to have an effect. Though this can pose a challenge when determining your dog's ideal dose. When the dose has been established and an administration routine perfected, sublingual cannabis is an excellent way to ensure your dog gets the cannabinoids it needs every time quickly and efficiently.

Topical Cannabis

There are patches, gels, and topical creams for use directly on the skin. Most topical cannabis will not cause a high, making them an excellent choice for delivering localized symptom relief.

They work quickly—between five to 15 minutes on average—by activating the CB2 receptors found in the pores and hair follicles of the skin. Researchers from the International Cannabinoid Research Society note the important role cannabinoid receptors play in the management of localized pain, inflammation, and dermatological health, and suggest that the application of supplemental cannabinoids such as those found in cannabis can help regulate these responses. Again, it is recommended that dog owners use hemp-based cannabis, which is very low in THC.

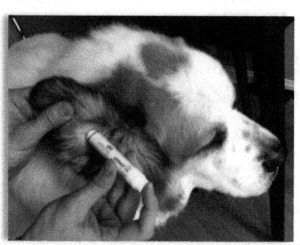

Topical CBD can be applied directly to the skin where dog cannot lick.

To be effective, cannabinoids must be extracted from the cannabis plant using either lipids—oils or alcohol. The cannabinoid-rich trichomes in the plant are not water soluble. So, to make cannabis topicals, either oil or alcohol is used to extract the cannabinoids from the plant.

Oil-Based Topicals: Oil-based topicals are the most popular CBD product on the market today. The oil used may be coconut or hemp oil, both of which are shown to improve elasticity, resilience, and many other dermatological conditions. Oil-based topicals can reduce pain and inflammation, treat topical conditions like psoriasis and allergies, and stimulate hair follicles.

It should be noted that oil-based topicals tend to stay on the skin surface, which can irritate your dog. Preventing your dog from licking the topical ointment can be tricky. Because licking is a common reaction to stress in dogs, applying weed-based topical ointments to a paw could cause a cycle of stress-induced licking. So be careful and watch your dog closely when using oil-based cannabis topicals.

Alcohol-based Topicals: Alternatively, cannabinoids may be extrated into alcohol, which can then be used to make topical products. Though not as popular as oil-based topicals because of their tendency to dry the skin—especially through repeated use, alcohol-based topicals tend to absorb into CB receptors more quickly while leaving virtually no residue on the skin surface. When it comes to topical canine treatment, alcohol-based cannabis topicals are very beneficial because they offer relief quickly without prompting your dog into heavy licking.

Alcohol-based cannabis topicals may be more potent because fewer complementary ingredients need to be added. Highly concentrated alcohol topicals are ideal for applying to tumors or other abnormal growths on the skin surface, though lotion may be needed to keep the skin from drying out or becoming overly irritated by repeated applications.

When applying topical cannabis to dogs, it's important that the product comes into direct con-

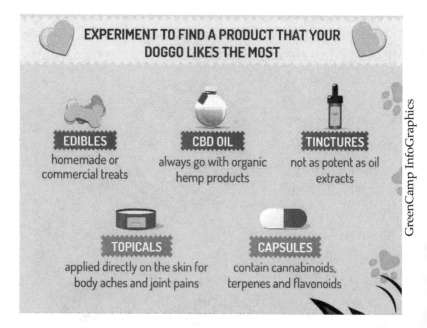

EXPERIMENT TO FIND A PRODUCT THAT YOUR DOGGO LIKES THE MOST

EDIBLES
homemade or commercial treats

CBD OIL
always go with organic hemp products

TINCTURES
not as potent as oil extracts

TOPICALS
applied directly on the skin for body aches and joint pains

CAPSULES
contain cannabinoids, terpenes and flavonoids

GreenCamp InfoGraphics

tact with the skin. For best results, the area should be shaved, clean, and left alone for at least five to fifteen minutes. Discourage your dog from licking the product from its skin by wrapping it in a bandage, using a cone or recovery collar, or simply petting your dog while the topicals take effect.

Suppositories

Rectal ingestion of cannabis is great for a few reasons: it absorbs quickly into the bloodstream and nearby organs, and it significantly reduces the likelihood of developing any sort of "high," even when high doses of THC are involved.

Cannabis suppositories are especially beneficial for dogs with urinary or digestive issues, and those suffering cancer, especially if the cancer cells reside in the digestive tract, because they allows consumption of very concentrated amounts of cannabinoids without the unpleasant side effects.

It's important to note that rectal and vaginal cannabis suppositories are different products. Whereas

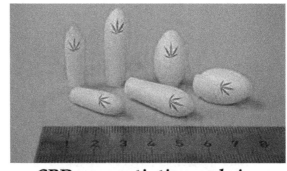

CBD suppostioties are being developed for dogs.

rectal cannabis suppositories can deliver up to 90 percent of its cannabinoid content directly to the blood and surrounding tissue, vaginal suppositories also contain a carrier agent to help them break the blood-brain barrier.

There are currently few cannabis suppositories on the market for dogs, largely due to dosing discrepancies and lesser demand for the product. However, given the popularity of cannabis suppositories in European countries coupled with America's love for anything weed-related, dog pot suppositories will likely soon be available to the general public.

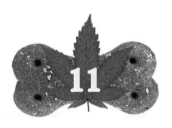

Dosing

Dosing is the trickiest part of using cannabis for canines. Medicinal cannabis for humans can be *very* potent and should *not* be used with dogs. Especially worrisome is the THC content, because dogs, in particular, react more strongly to THC than do we humans. For this reason it is better to stick with hemp-based products, especially when beginning to use cannabis with your dog, because hemp has very low levels of THC content so there is little risk of toxicity.

CBD has no toxic level so it is safe to give to your dog. Always follow the instructions on the packaging. But don't worry if you give your dog too much. It won't hurt your dog. You'll just be wasting the CBD.

Dosing depends upon many factors, most importantly including the type of product, your dog's weight, and the aliment being treated.

Dosing is the trickiest part of using cannabis for canines

Type of Product

CBD Oil: Given in drops. Generally give 2-4 drop, 2-4 times a day.

Capsule: Usually contain 150-200mg extract each. Give 1 cap 1-2 times day.

Treats: Vary in concentration. Always follow instructions on package.

Your dog's weight is important in dosing. Heavier dogs get a higher dose. Always follow instrucitons on the package.

Dose for Hemp-based CBD Oils

Small Dogs - under 20 lbs
2-3 drops, 3-4 times daily

Large Dogs - over 20 lbs
3-4 drops, 3-4 times daily

Biphasic Dosing Curve

The effects of medicinal cannabis follow a biphasic dosing curve, which looks like what we call "the normal curve". The horizontal line at the bottom is strength of dose. The vertical line on the left the intensity of effect. The optimal dose is at the peak of the curve—a kind of "sweet spot", while a smaller dose or a greater dose is less effective.

A study of the biphasic dose window at the University of Chicago looked at people who had used cannabis before but were not regular users. It showed that 7.5 mg of THC induced a mild elevation of mood and sense of well-being, while 12.5 mg of THC made subjects anxious. The challenge in dosing is finding that sweet spot for *your* dog. Healing with cannabis is more shaman-like than medical. Dosing is very individualized; each animal reacts a little differently. The rule of thumb is to "start low; go slow"—especially with any product containing THC.

The challenge in dosing is finding that sweet spot for your dog.

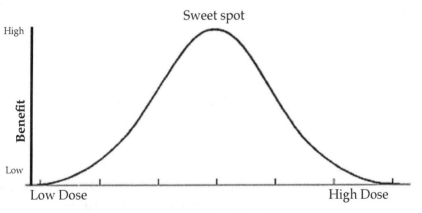

Biphasic Dosing Curve

Generally, for humans, products are made from a ratio of CBD to THC that makes up the total amount of CBD + THC—in milligrams—in a given dose. Dog owners should use hemp-based cannabis, which is very low in THC. However,

THC does have its benefits for dogs but MUST be introduced *very slowly* under guidance of a vet.

Look for products that have the ratio in milligrams on the label. Oakland Integrative vet, Dr. Gary Richter says you need to have the actual milligrams of CBD and THC—not just the ratio—for accurate dosing. Never use medicinal cannabis meant for humans on your dog, without specific guidance from a vet.

CBD : THC Ratios

High CBD [4-30 mg] : Low THC [1 mg]

examples 30:1; 20:1; 5:1

Equal CBD [1 mg] : THC [1mg]

example 1:1

Low CBD [1 mg] : High THC [4-20 mg]

examples 1:5; 1:10; 1:20

High THC Ratios

Smoke, tinctures, and edible forms of cannabis commonly have high THC content because it is used for recreation. Dog owners must be most careful of products for humans with high THC. because of the high risk of toxicity.

While it is advised that dog owners use hemp-based cannabis with their dog because of its low

THC—less than .03 mg. Dr Richter does provide information on calculating THC dosage for dogs—for educational purposes and not as advice.

To calculate a safe dose you must know the exact milligram concentration of the THC and CBD in a dose, which should be on the label. You should consult with a very knowledgeable vet to guide you, which is another challenge because vets are prohibited by law from recommending or dispensing cannabis.

Applications

High CBD : Low THC is good for GI issues, anxiety, pain, seizures, GI Problems, behavior problems and restlessness. Risk of toxicity is low because of the low THC content. Dog owners can generally use hemp-based safely because it has the highest CBD : THC ratio, with 25 to 1 to 25 or 30 to 1.

Equal Ratios: A twice daily dose of equal ratio of CBD to THC is generally used for neurologic disease, brain/spinal trauma, cancer, pain, inflammatory GI distress.

Low CBD : High THC is generally used for severe pain, Cancer, appetite, cancer.

Dosing Strategy—Titrate

Finding your dog's optimal dose takes titrating, a continuous measuring and adjusting of the dose, while monitoring the effects. No matter the condition being treated, *always start on a low THC dose product and slowly increase the amount of THC given—as needed.* Increase on weekly basis. Don't rush because your dog's body must adapt to the THC in order to tolerate it to limit possible toxicity, so that the THC can do its magic.—to allow to develop tolerance and limit possible toxicity.

Cautions

Make sure to consult your vet if your dog is taking *any* pharmaceutical. Cannabis has been known to potentiate—increase the power—of pharmaceuticals.

Remember, your furry pet can't tell you with words how it feels, so you must be careful to go slow and to monitor your dog's responses.

How to Calculate a Dose:

Dr. Gary Richter, author of *The Ultimate Pet Health Guide,* has a formula for figuring out low and high doses of THC and CBD. Despite the restrictions on vets to recommend cannabis, vets like Dr. Richter believe that it is important that dog owners have information upon which to make

Healing with cannabis is more shaman-like than medical.

good choices in treatment. Free Speech is the pro-tective veil Dr. Richter uses. He gives information to education under his free speech right.

Medicinal cannabis has been decriminalized for human use in various states, but in no case has it been decriminalized for dogs. With that disclaimer said, here is the careful, conservative formula for identifying your dog's individualized dose.

Weigh Your Dog

The amount of dose is based upon your dog's weight—in kilograms. So the first step is to weigh your dog and then to convert it from pounds to kilograms. **One kilogram is equal to 2.2 pounds.** So you divide your dog's weight in pounds by 2.2 to get its weight in kilograms.

Weight Conversion

1 Kilogram (kg) = 2.2 pounds
Weight in kgs x 2.2 = weight in lbs
Weight in pounds / 2.2 = weight in kgs

Dosing Range

Remember *Start low; Go slow* is how you titrate up to the optimal dose. Here is the dosing range from low to high.

THC dosing range: 0.1 to 0.25 mg/kg per day = 0.05 to 0.125 given twice a day.

CBD dosing range: 0.1 to 0.5 mg/kg per day = 0.05 to 0.25 given twice a day.

Since doses are generally given twice a day, those amount would then be divided by 2 to get the mg/per dose.

Steps to Calculating Dose

Now with the above data in hand you can calculate the individualized dose for your dog.

Steps to Calculate Dose

1. Convert weight from pounds to kilograms
2. Multiply weight in kilograms by THC low dose [0.1]
3. Multiply weight in kilogram by THC high dose. [0.25]
4. Multiply weight in kilogram by CBD low dose [0.1]
5. Multiply weight in kilograms by CBD high dose [0.5

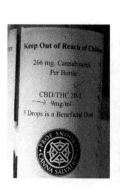
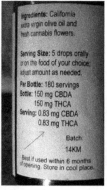
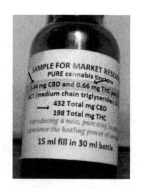

To calculate a safe dose you must know the exact milligram concentration of the THC and CBD.

6. Divide #2-#3 calc mil THC by # mg in the medicine
   [mil per drop, per dropper, etc]
7. Divide #4-#5 calc mil CBD by # mg in the medicine
8. Divide #6-#7 by 2 to get am and pm daily doses.

An Example

Lil Lu
15 pound Jack Russell
Tincture potency:

   1.44 mg CBD: 0.66 mg THC per drop

1. Lil Lu's weight in kilograms is 15/2.2 =
   6.82 kilograms rounded to 6.8 kg.
2. Low THC dose is 6.8 x 0.1 = .68 mil;
3. High THC dose is 6.8 x 0.25 = 1.7 mg
4. Low CBD dose is 6.8 x 0.1 = .68 mil;
5. High CBD dose is 6.8 x 0.5 = 3.4 mil.
6. Low THC .68/0.66 = 1.030 = 1 mg;
   High THC 1.7/0.66 = 2.575 = 2.6 mg.
7. Low CBD .68/1.44 = .4722 = .47 mg;
   High CBD 3.4 mg/1.44 mg = 2.361 = 2.6 mg
8. Low THC 1/2 = .5 am/pm;
   High THC 1.7 mg/2 = .85 mg am/pm
   Low CBD .47/2 = .235 = .23 mg am/pm
   High CBD 2.6/2 = 1.3 mg am/pm

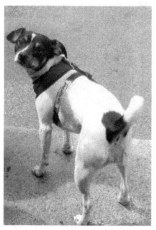

Lil Lu's am/pm Dose
Low
.23 CBD : .5 THC.
High
1.3 CBD : 2.3 THC

Lil Lu

Retail Product Dosing

With the prohibitions on vets and the ongoing illegal status of cannabis for dogs, and resulting lack of research, getting reliable dosing information is difficult. Budtenders in dispensaries may be helpful in giving information for human use, but are not likely to be too knowledgeable about use with dogs. Manufacturers of cannabis products for dogs is another source of helpful information. King Kanine is one such company and is recommended by Brian Armstrong of the *Cannabis for Pets Blog*.

King Kanine offers CBD:THC tinctures in a variety of strengths: 75mg/30ML, 150mg/30ML, and 300mg/30ML.They provide a helpful weight x dosing table for each tincture. Shown here is the dosing chart for King Kanine 300mg/30ML CBD.

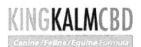

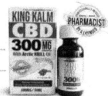

KING**KALM**CBD

Canine/Feline/Equine Formula

Please check our website for updated Lab Tests and product information. www.kingkanine.com

A Natural **Cannabidiol** Product

Dosage chart for

300mg/30ML

Canine and Feline Formula's

Dog/Cats Weight (LBS)	STANDARD	THERAPEUTIC	MEDICINAL
5	.1ml	.1ml	.2ml
10	.1ml	.1ml	.3ml
15	.2ml	.2ml	.4ml
20	.2ml	.3ml	.5ml
25	.2ml	.4ml	.75ml
30	.3ml	.4ml	1ml
35	.4ml	.4ml	1ml
40	.4ml	.5ml	1ml
45	.5ml	.6ml	1.75ml
50	.5ml	.8ml	2ml
55	.5ml	.8ml	2ml
60	.5ml	.8ml	2ml
65	.6ml	.9ml	2ml
70	.6ml	.9ml	2.5ml
75	.7ml	1ml	2.5ml
80	.7ml	1ml	3ml
85	.8ml	1ml	3ml
90	1ml	1.5ml	3ml
95	1ml	1.5ml	3.2ml
100	1ml	1.7ml	3.3ml
101-120	1ml	1.8ml	3.5ml
121-140	1ml	2ml	3.5ml
141-160	1.2ml	2ml	3.75ml

½ .5ml
1 1.1
½ 1.6ml
2 2.1
½ 2.6
3 ml

Use the same dose structure for both dogs and cats.

To Dose: Read the info on the back to determine how to dose. How to: Simply fill the provided syringe with the amount you have chosen based on a daily or situational administration as it pertains to your dog or cats need. Put the empty oral syringe over the tip on the open bottle and extract the amount desired. Rinse syringe and use for future dosing.

• **Standard:** General immune/health support. Situational ie: separation, thunderstorms, travel, crowds, during grooming or any situation that may cause anxiety.
• **Therapeutic:** Anxiety, Arthritis, Inflammation, Hip Dysplasia, Nausea or Vomiting, Pain from injury or post surgery
• **Medicinal:** Cancers, Epilepsy, Hip Dysplasia or any situation that may cause a need for higher dosing amounts.

This product has not been approved by the FDA and is not intended to treat, diagnose, or cure any disease. Always consult a physician prior to supplementing any product.

KING KANINE
PET WELLNESS **INSIDE** AND **OUT**

www.kingkanine.com

Notice , like in Dr. Richter's approach, King Kaine specifies three levels of treatment: Standard, Therapeutic, and Medicinal.

Levels of Treatment

Standard: General immune & health support, situational anxiety from noise, travel, crowds, separation, during grooming.

Therapeutic: Anxiety, arthritis, inflammation, hip dysplasia, nausea or vomiting, pain from injury or joint pain.

Medicinal: Cancers, epilepsy, hip dysplasia, or any situation that may cause a need for a higher dosing amounts.

Besides the helpful detailed dosing chart for each product, King Kaine provides a syringe for accurately measuring the dose.

Dosing Instructions

Always be cautious. Begin at the low end of the dose range and increase slowly once weekly to enable your dog's body to adjust to the THC. *Slow is the rule.* Allow at least 3-4 weeks to move from the low end to the high end of the dose while tracking effects.

Remember: Because of the biphasic dosing curve, the most optimal dose for your dog will probably be less than your highest calculated dose. Monitor signs of loss of balance, excessive sedation, or abnormal behavior that might be indication of too much THC. Contact your veterinarian immediately if you see anything concerning.

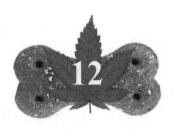

How to Medicate Your Dog

Giving medicine to dogs can be difficult, especially when they so obviously don't like it. Following your veterinarian's prescription recommendation precisely is important to helping your furry pal have the best outcome possible. When administering medication to your dog, there are a few things you should remember.

Administering Pills and Capsules

The most common form of medication prescribed to dogs is pills and capsules. Though some dog owers may be lucky enough to simply wrap it in a slice of cheese and hand it over, more often than not, a little more convincing is required to see that the medication makes it to your dog's stomach where it can do its thing.

Your veterinarian will show you the correct procedure for pill administration, and will probably make it look incredibly easy, too. Remember, vets have had a lot of practice with the process and still struggle sometimes. Don't give up! It is imperative that your dog receives the medication the veterinarian prescribed at the proper time and proper dose.

Grinding up your dog's pills is a big no-no, because doing so can affect the dose and the potency of the medication. Tablets have a protective coating to protect them from dissolving too fast. If a pill is ground up before administering, it may dissolve too quickly, some may get lost during consumption, rendering the medication to be less effective.

Administering Liquids Meds

In some cases such as when dealing with small animals like puppies, liquid oral medication may be recommended. As with pills, your veterinarian will show you exactly how to administer the liquid medications using the included eyedropper as a measuring tool.

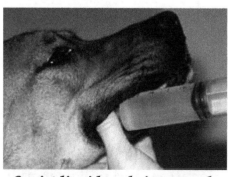

Squirt liquid meds into pouch between the cheek and teeth.

Liquid medications often require special storage or preparation. For example, some liquid medications need to be stored in the refrigerator to keep them at optimum potency while others may separate and settle if held on a shelf too long. Before administering the liquid medication, roll the product between your palms—rather than shaking it—to mix without creating air bubbles which can render the dose inaccurate.

Administering Topical Medications

Topical meds are probably the least traumatizing form of medicine administration, but that doesn't mean there are no challenges involved, specifically, how to keep your pooch from licking the medicine off! Giving your dog a tasty treat may suffice long enough for the medication to take effect. Try a treat that requires some licking of its own such as peanut butter or canned dog food because those foods take more time to finish.

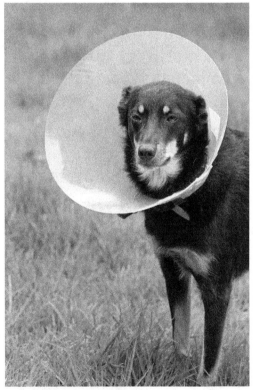

Dog wearing Queen Anne collar.

If the licking continues a "Queen Anne Collar" may be

required. Your veteterinarial will probaly provide you with a cone—or "recovery"—collar during your appointment, but if not, you can buy one inexpensively at your local pet store or online.

How to Give Your Dog a Pill

Hold the dog's head from the top using your left hand if you are right-handed. If the dog has a long nose hold the upper jaw between thumb and index finger.

Tilt the dog's head back. Gently fold the upper lip over the teeth as you open the mouth so that if the dog bites down with your hand in its mouth, it will bite its lip, not your hand. Place your thumb on the roof of the dog's mouth.

Hold the pill in your right hand between your thumb and index finger. Use the middle finger of your right hand to pull open the lower jaw. Keep your middle finger over the small incisor teeth *not* over the sharp canine teeth.

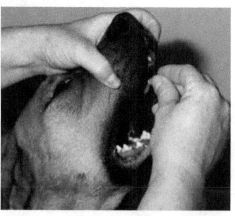

Push the pill as far back over the tongue as possible so that it over the throat. If you are unable to get the pill far enough over the base of the

Hold the dog's head from the top.

tongue, the dog will spit it out. Immediately close the dog's mouth and rub its throat, which will encourage it to swallow.

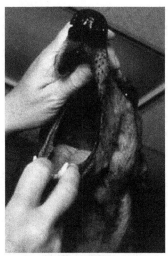

For liquid medications squirt the medication into the pouch between the teeth and cheek. Then hold your dog's mouth closed the mouth and stroke the throat to encourage the dog to swallow.

Pull dog's lip over upper teeth to avoid being bitten.

Liquids are more likely to accidentally enter the windpipe compared to pills or capsules. *Do not* tilt the dog's head backward to avoid the dog inhaling liquid into the windpipe,.

If you find it difficult to give your dog a pill or capsule, speak to your veterinarian about suspending the pill or capsule in a liquid. Some medications can be suspended in liquid while others lose their effectiveness when placed in a suspension. Always talk to your veterinarian before modifying any medication regime.

We want to keep our family members happy and healthy for a long, long time—all of them— which sometimes requires a bit of medical intervention. But when it comes to medicating dogs,

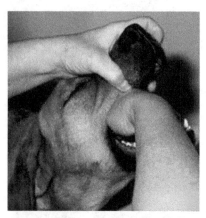

Push pill to the back of the dog's throat.

the different drug types, short and long term effects, careful dosing instructions and dangerous drug interactions can be confusing. Though we never recommend deviating from your veterinarian's recommendations, there may be an alternative—or a boost—for sometimes harsh prescription pet medications.

Monitoring Treatment

With the recent legalization of cannabis around the nation, dog owners wonder about medicating their furry friends with cannabis. Research on cannabis for canines is extremely limited, and even anecdotal evidence is hard to discern. For example, even though no human has ever fatally overdosed on cannabis consumption, safety for dogs is less clear.

While dog and human Endocannanbinoid Systems function the same, cannabinoids have a more profound impact on dogs due to their smaller size and faster metabolic rate. As with humans, individual dogs vary in their sensitivity to cannabinoids.

It is our responsibility as the loving dog owner to dose properly as well as to monitor symptoms, doses, frequency, and so on.

How Monitoring Helps

- You discover the best cannabis therapy practices for your dog; and

- Your veterinarian can better evaluate how cannabinoid intervention is helping your dog live the happy life it deserves.

Determining Symptoms

Your dog can't tell you when it's feeling ill or otherwise uncomfortable, so it's important to watch its mannerisms to notice changes in behavior. If you notice new behaviors, like excessive licking, urinary incontinence, changes in appetite, and other changes, pull out a pen and notepad and start monitoring, i.e., count the behavior to determine its frequency. Doing so can help you iden-

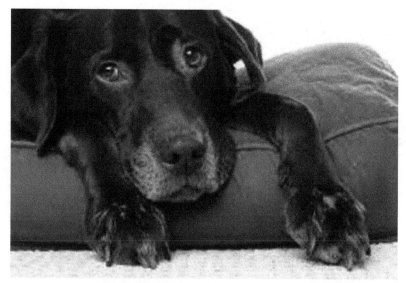

Observe your dog closely for symptoms of distress.

tify the problem quickly, determine a treatment option, and ensure treatment is working to get Fido back on the road to optimum health.

There is a long list of potential symptoms your dog could display to let you know he or she isn't up to par. Again, it's up to you to notice symptoms and monitor them to determine the severity and best plan of action.

Symptoms of Canine Distress

- Fear of loud noises
- Bad breath
- Gas
- Drooling
- Hair loss
- Dry or flaky skin
- Constipation or diarrhea
- Excessive licking/scratching
- Bumps, ulcers or lesions under the skin
- Limping
- Sneezing
- Vomiting
- Red eyes
- Rapid weight change
- Altered eating habits

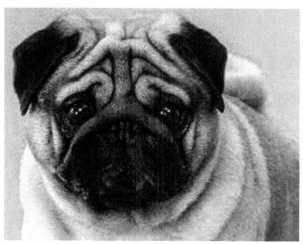

Ravin

Though some of these symptoms, like gas, could seem like no more than a simple annoyance, it could be the sign of a bigger issue. Monitoring symptoms and seeking quick treatment could save your pooch—and you—a lot of trouble and heart ache in the long run.

For example, Shirley has two dogs, a 12-year-old pug named Ravin and a five-year-old Husky/Chow mix named Charlie. Shortly after adopting Charlie, little Ravin began urinating in the house. At first, Shirley thought Ravin was peeing in the house because of Charlie often peed at the door because she thought it was okay or maybe it was a territorial response.

Shirley attempted to re-train little Ravin to go potty outside. But Ravin knew she was supposed to go outside because she still asked to go out when she had to pee, but often, it seemed she didn't even bother to try.

Shirley kept trying to retrain Ravin to go outside as she followed Ravin around cleaning up her offensive-smelling surprises around the house. Then Shirley came across an article on-line that reported urinary incontinence is a common symptom of a hormonal imbalance in dogs.

Armed with information, Shirley took Ravin to the vet to discover she had developed "Spay Incontinence" characterized by a weakened urethral sphincter following the spaying process. The vet told Shirley that approximately 20 percent of female dogs develop the disorder within three years of being spayed, with the likeliness and severity increasing with age. Using a combination of estrogen therapy and non-hormonal medications, Ravin has been able to keep her "go" to herself until she's able to dispel it outside.

Other symptoms are just as important to monitor closely, including how quickly the symptoms came about, how frequently they occur and so on. For example, though the cause of diarrhea could be something as simple as a change in diet, it could also be a sign of a bacteria, viral, or parasitic infection. Your veterinarian will need to know if the volume of stool is more or

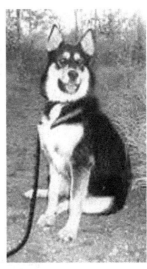

Charlie

less than what is common, if your dog strained to pass the stool, if there was any blood or mucus present, if vomiting accompanies diarrhea and so on. When monitoring your dog's symptoms, record every detail to report to your vet.

Monitor your dog's diet while monitoring symptoms. Your dog may experience an increase or decrease in thirst or appetite, or may have an aversion to an ingredient in its food.

What to Monitor for Food Intake

- The time the food was consumed
- The total amount of food eaten
- The brand/source of the food
- Your dog's apparent level of hunger/thirst

Other things to monitor include weight, which should be measured every two months, is especially important for senior dogs. For smaller breeds, you can do this by weighing yourself, then picking up your dog and weighing both of you then subtracting the difference to arrive at your dog's weight. Larger dogs may require the use of a veterinarian's scale. Record the weight bi-monthly and report drastic changes to your veterinarian immediately.

Note changes in your dog's behavior. Has its sleeping pattern changed? Is it less attentive to commands? Is your dog easily startled or does it act anxious when you're about to leave?

Monitor motor activity, such as difficulty climbing stairs, exercise without exhaustion, or bumping into things when walking. These could be symptoms of neurological disorders, arthritis, or glaucoma, all of which are more likely in dogs over the age of 10 years.

Count frequency of behavior/symptom

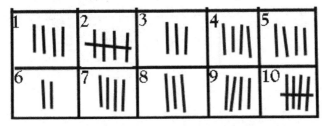

Count the number of times that the symptom occurs within a specific time, such as 10 5-minute samples.

Finally, watch for skin abnormalities during grooming and petting. Check for lumps, abrasions, bald spots, redness, or other concerns. Make note of any symptoms, along with the size at the time of discovery, the texture or consistency, and whether or not your dog seems to be irritated by them. Skin abnormalities could have a range of causes—from dander in the grass to anxiety or even cancer—so it's important to monitor the characteristics of the abnormality closely.

Counting

A good way to monitor is to count the frequency of the behavior or symptom being monitored. Especially when the symptom is happening frequently, it is difficult to see small improvements

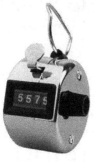

because it keeps occuring so often. Counting and comparing shows changes. For example, perhaps your dog scratches a lot. You count the number of time it scratches in specific 15 minute periods through out the day.

Counter

Using a golf counter to record the frequency of your dog's symptom, such as biting its back, makes counting easy. There are two types. A hand-held counter and wrist counter, like a watch, that you wear on your wrist. When you see your dog biting its back, you press the counter which records it. You don't have to keep remembering the number. Just click. Later record the total count for a particular time sample on a chart. Seeing the "data" visually helps to make it understandable. Makes seeing progress, or its lack, easy.

When counting before starting treatment such as giving your dog a tincture

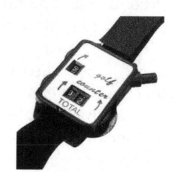

Wrist counter

of hemp CBD for it's skin as a treatment for its scratching. The count before treatment is the "baseline", which is measured before intervention begins. The baseline count, compared to later count after intervention, gives a starting point to measure effectiveness of the intervention.

Rating

Another way to monitor and gather a baseline is with ratings. Some behaviors/symptom occur as a matter of degree such as excitability, lethergy, apparent anxiety. Here it can be useful to use a scale such as 1 to 9, where 1 is low in the behavior such as very calm and 9 is extremely excited. Then you would observe your dog and rate it's

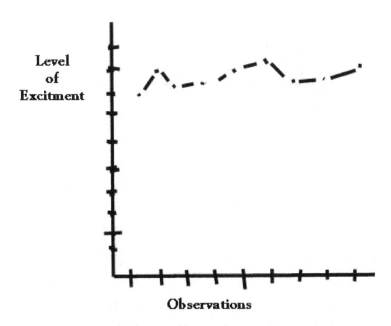

Rate the degree of the behavior or symptom, then plot rating on a chart.

level of excitment somewhere between 1 and 9. It helps to use a odd number because then there is a middle, which in this example is 5. Ratings are plotted on a chart.

Determining Treatment Effectiveness

Though monitoring symptoms will help determine the cause of them, without bloodwork or

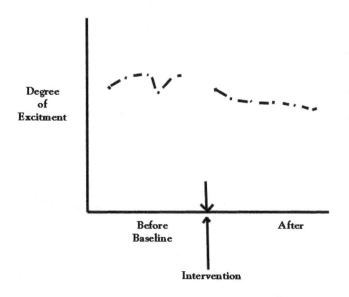

Continue to rate and plot after intervention to see effectiveness of treatment.

extensive testing, it may be difficult to diagnose your dog's problems. After monitoring your dog's symptoms and deciding on a treatment option with your vet, add another column—or

two or three
depending on
the number of
medical inter-

*Most veterinarians are still unable
to recommend cannabis therapy
for legal reasons.*

ventions recommended by your vet—to your
monitoring sheet to help monitor the success
of treatment. This should include the treatment
method itself, the dose (if applicable), the frequency of administration, and notes regarding
the administration process.

Continue to monitor all other symptoms
during the treatment process because it helps determine whether or not the treatment is effective.

Be Systematic

The best way to determine if a treatment is effective is to use the scientific method to monitor your dog's progress. For example, if you've
noticed that your dog gets anxious at the sound
of the vacuum, you can try different methods to
reduce its anxiety and monitor which are effective.
Administer the intervention, record details regarding the administration, then note whether or not
the symptoms improve, the extent to which they
improved, and how long it took for you to be able
to detect the improvement. If no noticeable improvement is detected, record that, as well.

Some people have successfully treated anxiety in dogs with music therapy—soothing music

works best, synthetic pheromones, sedatives, or even a good ol' pet-down using a dryer sheet to eliminate static electicity. Sometimes static electricity in the carpets causes dog to get anxious. It is not "all or nothing". CBD has been shown to reduce anxiety and work well in combination with other medications, as well.

Determining Benefits of Supplementation

In addition to your veterinarian recommended treatment options, you may choose to supplement your dog with cannabinoids like CBD or CBN. Before beginning cannabis therapy, discuss your plan with your vet and decide together on the best mode of action. Your vet may not be able to recommend cannabis therapy due to licensing restrictions, but should support your decision and work with you to determine if the effectiveness of the cannabis treatment

When introducing cannabis therapy to your dog, first determine the symptoms that need to be addressed using the simple monitoring method discussed earlier. After you've charted your dog's symptoms, compare them alongside a list of cannabinoids and their benefits.

Giving your dog THC should be avoided because it is toxic to dogs—except when introduced very slowly. Most products for dogs are made from hemp oil which has less than .3% THC and was recently partially legalized across the nation with the Farm Act of 2014. Look for cannabis products that contain the "full spectrum" of cannabinoids and terpenes. Research shows that CBD alone is not as effective as it is when working in unison with other cannabinoids. Terpenes give the cannabinoid's effects some depth which adds to the therapeutic value.

Due to the illegality of cannabis at the federal level, only certain products may be legal in your area. Cannabinoids derived from the hemp plant are generally legal and considered safe for administration—as opposed to extracts from the plant, *Cannabis Sativa L.*, a.k.a. "marijuana" which may contain traces of THC. Check the product labels for additives that may dilute the product, and check the ingredients for a complete list of cannabinoids.

Determine if the product is "full spectrum", which contains the "full spectrum" of cannabinoids and terpenes from the original plant or "isolate", which is just the flavorless, colorless crystals of individual cannabinoids like CBD. Having a clear understanding of the total cannabinoid profile administered to your pet will help you and your vet determine which—if any—cannabinoids are the most beneficial to your dog.

Though CBD alone provides numerous benefits to the body—pain relief, anti-inflammation, anti-anxiety, neuroprotection, etc.—there are some things it simply cannot do. If your dog needs help falling asleep, for example, it may benefit from the cannabinoid, CBN, which has been shown to promote sleep in humans. Likewise, cannabinoids like CBC or CBG are better for treating fungal infections.

Anxiety & Stress

Anxious dogs often inappropriately urinate or defecate, tremble, try to escape, chew things, dig, and lick excessively. If your dog exhibits a lot of anxiety symptoms, CBD can help to relieve and soothe them. The first step is to identify the anxiety trigger before starting supplementation. Separation anxiety is the second most common behavior problem of canines affecting an estimated 14% to 40% of dogs. Dogs are pack animals and may experience separation anxiety when left alone. Mixed breeds may be more prone to separation anxiety than purebred dogs and male dogs may be at higher risk than females. In addition to separation anxiety, these dogs may have other panic disorders or phobias including nighttime panic.

Dogs can also experience situational anxiety in crowds, when traveling, and around loud noise, such as from firecrackers, and thunder. More seriously, dogs that have been physically or mentally abused often have specific phobias and fears and are prone to experiencing free-floating anxiety.

Because dogs are very in tune with their environment, sudden environmental changes can trigger anxiety. For example, moving into a new home can stress dogs, as can the arrival of a new family member or the presence of strangers or strange animals, or the death of a companion dog, as happened to Disney, my small whippet-mix who was the companion to Zoe, my beautiful brown pit. Zoe was a 16+ year-old senior when she suddenly died. Disney was very distressed. She sat in her bed looking at me sternly, as if to say, "Why are you abusing me? Where is Zoe?" She snubbed her meals, while continuing to stare at me. "Where is Zoe?" When I put food into her mouth—pufft—as she immediately spit it out, while quivering.

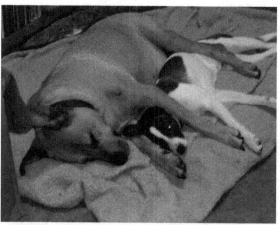

I didn't know about CBD for dogs, at the time. So instead on day ten, I went to shelters and then hit Craigslists looking for a puppy for Disney,

Disney became extremely anxious when her companion, Zoe, died.

Then I drove to a woman's apartment, gave her one hundred bucks, and came away with Lil Lu. I felt guilty getting another dog when my beautiful Zoe had only been gone less than 2 weeks.

Disney wasn't pleased. She lay in her bed staring darts at Lil Lu, sitting on my lap, as if to say, "Who is that punk?!!" Finally, after nearly 2 weeks of continued upset and distress, I called Disney over and said out loud, "Disney, if you don't like Lil Lu, we can take her back." Amazingly, Disney looked at me, jumped down and got into the dog bed with Lil Lu. They have been fast friends ever since!

Signs of Anxiety

- Panting
- Pacing
- Whimpering
- Trembling
- Fidgeting
- Barking
- Aggresison
- Peeing
- Destructive chewing

Employing distraction strategies is common to reduce separation anxiety in dogs when leaving them alone. For example, dog owners may give

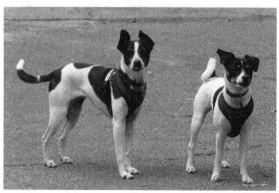

their nervous pooch a bone as a distraction when leaving home to reduce the likelihood of their dog chewing up their shoes.

Disney and Lil Lu are best friends.

Anxious canine behaviors are not the result of disobedience or spite. Your dog displays anxious behaviors when left alone because it's upset and trying to cope with and adapt to a great deal of stress! This is where CBD can be very helpful for anxious dogs.

CBD has been shown to help gently and effectively reduce anxiety. It can be added to a daily health regimen or used as needed, such as prior to road trip, for example, to help your dog stay calm. Always follow the dosing instructions on the product packaging.

Alicia's dog Hudson, an 80 pound shepherd mix, was generally anxious especially around strangers and loud noises. Friends were coming to stay over the 4th of July weekend. Alicia expected that Hudson would be nervous so she decided to try some commercial CBD dog treats she bought at a pet store. The packaging recommended 1 treat for each 40 lbs, twice daily. So Alicia gave Hudson 2 treats, which he loved and scarfed right down. Watching Hudson, Alicia reported, "After about 30-45 minutes I noticed Hudson became more relaxed, but not lethargic or out of it. He simply didn't start barking or growling at every noise he heard outside like he normally does throughout the day."

Cheryl's Black Lab, Cupid, was only 6 weeks old when she adoped him. Cupid was a great dog, trained quickly, and had no issues—until suddenly, at 5 years old, he became scared of fireworks. Cheryl tried all the tricks for situational anxiety. She bought him a compression shirt to help with 4th of July firreworks . "It did nothing," said Cheryl. "Cupid shredded my living room carpet."

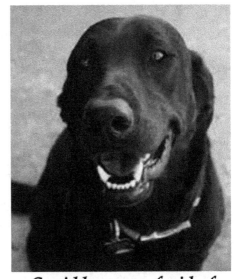

Soon his anxiety progressed to include thunderstorms. The anxiety meds from the vet did nothing. "I tried every 'calming' treat I could find. Nothing worked. One day a friend suggested she try CBD with Cupid. She didn't wait long

Cupid became afraid of fireworks and thumder.

to try it, because there was a huge thunderstorm the next week. "Cupid was so upset and terrified, I decided to try the oil. Within about 10-15 minutes, Cupid was laying by my feet on the couch as I listened to the storm rage outside. Cupid's response to the CBD was amazing."

Behavioral Anxiety

The soothing and calming action of CBD is helpful in reducing situational anxiety. On the other hand, behavioral anxiety, such as that triggered by phobia and fears, which suggests negative psychological conditioning, can't be "fixed" by using CBD alone. Behavioral problems, such as aggression like snapping, or excessive groveling and hiding, have probably been instilled—conditioned—by earlier abuse. Conditioning is another word for learning. When abused—punished—dogs learn phobias—fears—and dysfunctional behavior. Such ingrained anxiety responses can be un-learned and replaced with appropriate behavior through training with positive reinforcement.

Retraining anxiety responses takes skill, time, and patience. Teaching a dog to be calm rather than anxious is faster when the dog is calm during the training—which is a bit of a contradiction. If the dog could be calm during training to learn to be calm, it doesn't need the training; whereas an excessively anxious dog on the verge

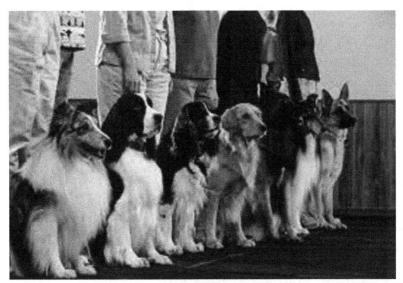

*A dose of CBD oil before training can facilitate
learning by calming your dog.*

of "hysterics" is not able to calm itself. Such a dog is "hardwired" for anxiety, which the smallest thing, like a loud noise, can turn on like a light switch. Here is where the soothing action of CBD can help.

CBD should be given to your dog about ½ to 1 hour before a train session to help your dog *to learn* to relax and *learn to* stay calm. Begin at the low end of dosing recommended on the product packaging and slowly increase it while monitoring your dog's apparent anxiety level during training, as well as following training.

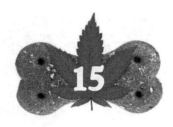

Pain & Inflammation

Watching your dog struggle with chronic pain is distressing. Pain and inflammation are caused by a range of conditions, from arthritis to a cut in a paw to pancreatitis. With our busy lives it is easy to overlook symptoms, especially since dogs can't speak up, but tend to suffer silently in the corner. It is important to be always monitoring your dog for signs of potential problems, so that you can take action before they become serious. That's why it's important to look out for signs of pain and treat the condition before it gets worst.

Inflammation is an immune response that is central to the body healing itself from infections and injury. The inflamed area turns red and becomes warm from the increased blood flow. Swelling and pressure is caused by blood vessels leaking fluid to the tissue surrounding the affected areas. Inflammation is a necessary part of the healing process. The problem is that with the swelling comes pain. Common inflammatory conditions include arthritis, bronchitis, colitis, and tonsillitis. Exterior injuries such as rashes, cuts, bites, dermatitis, skin conditions, ingrown nails, and sores cause pain and inflammation.

Inflammation shows itself as swelling and redness around the effected area. When joints are inflamed they become less mobile and may in-

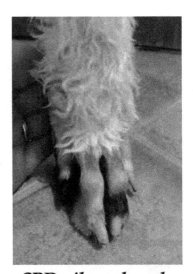

CBD oil can be rubbing into sores to soothe inflammation and speed healing.

clude mild limping or stiffness, weight gain, losing interest in playing, less alertness, and sleeping, difficulty jumping onto the bed and climbing up stairs.

CBD supplements can be administered twice daily—up to four times in extreme cases—for continued palliative relief from pain and discomfort. Both oral and topical applications can be effective. Swelling can be reduced by alternatively using ice pack on the swollen area for 10 minutes followed by heating pad on swollen area for 10 minutes. Then repeat 2-3 times an hour. Additional relief can be gained from rubbing a little of the CBD oil into the swollen area. In some

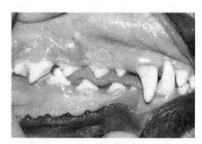

CBD oil appied with a Q-tip can soothe inflammed gums.

cases you may want to shave the area to expose your dog's skin, making it easier to rub CBD oil topically into the swollen area.

Inflammed gums can be relieved by using a Q-tip dipped into CBD oil and then rubbed onto your dog's gum.

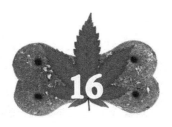

Gastrointestinal Upset

Signs of digestive system distress can include excessive drooling, diarrhea, constipation, vomiting, loss of appetite, bleeding, abdominal pain and bloating, shock, and dehydration. The location and nature of the distress often can be determined by the signs your dog shows. For example, abnormalities of biting, chewing, and swallowing usually are associated with diseases of the mouth, the teeth, the jaw, or the esophagus. Vomiting is usually due to inflammation of the lining of stomach or intestines—gastroenteritis—caused by infection or irritation. However, vomiting can also be caused by a non-digestive condition such as kidney disease.

Nausea is common in dogs. Your dog may vomit because it ate too much, too fast, or because it ate something uneatable. Dogs commonly eat grass when having an upset stomach. If your dog vomits more then once and appears sick, you should take it to the vet right away.

There are many causes of nausea in dogs and digestion issues. You can help your dog to purge its system by withholding food for 6 to 8 hours. During this fasting time you give it small amounts of water. After 10-12 hours of your dog not vomiting, give it a small meal of bland food such as white rice and boneless canned chicken meat. During the fasting, you might give your dog a few drops of CBD oil to help soothe its stomach.

Diarrhea is often a sign of digestive system disorders, but it can have many causes. Diarrhea can also be caused by mal-absorption, the failure to properly absorb nutrients.

Changes in the color, consistency, or frequency of feces are another sign of digestive problems. Black, tarry feces may be a sign of bleeding in the stomach or small intestine. Straining during bowel movements is usually associated with inflammation of the rectum and anus. Abdominal

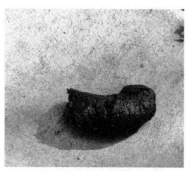

distention—bloating—can result from accumulation of gas, fluid, or ingested food, usually due to reduced activity of the muscles that move food through the digestive system. Distention can also be caused by a physical obstruction such as a

Tarry poop may indicate intestional bleeding.

foreign object or intussusception—"telescoping" of one part of the intestines into another, or from something as simple as overeating.

Vomiting

Dogs are a lot like kids. They're curious about everything and will put just about anything in their mouths. So, it's natural that your dog's curiosity can lead to some unexpected vomiting of foreign objects or food it ate too quickly. However, if you notice your dog vomiting frequently, or regurgitating undigested food accompanied by other signs of discomfort, a visit with your veterinarian is advised.

Some common reasons your dog may be vomiting include bacterial or viral infections, acute kidney or liver failure, pancreatitis, heat stroke, poisoning, or an adverse reaction to medication. Though cannabis cannot treat the causes of nausea, it can help make the sensations more bearable until you acquire the proper diagnosis and treatment.

Parasites are a frequent cause of digestive tract disorders in dogs. Many species of parasites can infect the digestive tract and cause disease. Parasites can cause severe disease or simply decrease your dog's overall fitness.

Danger Signs

- Blood in the vomit
- Dry heaving
- Bloated, swollen abdomen
- Dog ate something toxic
- Elevated temperature
- Gums are pale or yellow
- Dog is in pain
- Chronic diarrhea

Appetite Loss

Appetite loss, or anorexia as it's referred to in dogs, is often one of the first indications that your dog isn't feeling well. There may be a simple cause for your dog's appetite loss, such as a recent vaccination or a distaste for a new kind of food. However, when a dog doesn't eat, it's often an indication of a larger problem such as dental disease, anxiety, or pain, as examples. Consulting your veterinarian is recommended to diagnose the problem.

CBD supplements can improve appetite loss, when your dog learns to accept treats and tinctures. Common methods to encourage your dog to eat include adding fats, like bacon grease, to dry dog food, adding wet can food to your dog's dinner, heating the food, or making your dog's dinner from scratch using ingredients like rice; chicken or beef stock; protein like turkey or chicken; and vegetables like sweet potatoes, asparagus, spinach, carrots, and green beans. Add a few

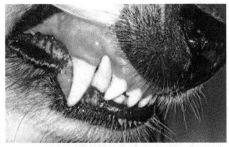

Apply CBD oil to gums about 10 minutes before dinner.

drops of CBD oil to your dog's food. Make sure to follow the dosing instructions on the product. Alternatively, you can apply a tincture to its gums about 10 minutes before dinner to allow the cannabinoids time to absorb into the bloodstream before eating.

Gastrointestinal Issues

Many digestive system diseases are not caused by infective organisms. Their causes include overeating, eating poor-quality food, chemicals, obstruction caused by swallowing foreign objects, or injury to the digestive system. Digestive system disease can also be caused by enzyme deficiencies, damage to the digestive tract such as from gastric ulcers, or birth defects. Digestive system signs such as vomiting and diarrhea may also occur because of kidney, liver, or adrenal gland disease.

Gastrointestinal disorders mean more than an achy stomach for your pooch. If your dog can't

digest its food properly, it could become dehy-
drated, malnourished, and dizzy as a result of
electrolyte imbalance. There are many types of
gastrointestinal diseases in dogs that occur frequently in breeds like German Shepherds, Collies,
Great Danes, and Golden Retrievers. While some
bouts may be short lived—after ingesting poisonous plants or foreign objects, for example—others
like colitis or pancreatitis will require medical
intervention.

Symptoms of gastrointestinal problems include vomiting, diarrhea, bloody stools, abdominal pain, weight loss, and lethargy, and should
clear up on their own within a few days. In the
meantime, you can give your dog a dose of CBD
tincture or oil twice daily. CBD can help reduce
pain and inflammation related to GI disorders
and can improve appetite, too.

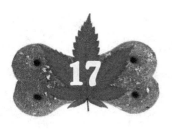

Allergies & Skin Problems

Your dog constantly licking may be a sign of something serious. The cause may anxiety or physical discomfort—like a burr stuck in the skin, or it may be a symptom of allergies, hormonal imbalances, or parasite infestation, such as with fleas and ticks.

Allergies are the leading cause of itchy skin. Almost 20% of the dogs suffer from itching, excessive hair loss, eczema or allergy. Forty percent of vet visits for skin problems are for itchy skin, which known as *pruritus*. One of the most common skin disease affecting dogs is *atopic dermatitis*, a chronic inflammatory disease associated with allergies. Dogs commonly suffer from three types of allergies: Allergies from fleas & mites, allergies from the environment—dust, plants, pollen, and mold, and food allergies.

Dogs can have an allergic reaction when their immune system becomes overactive and treats a

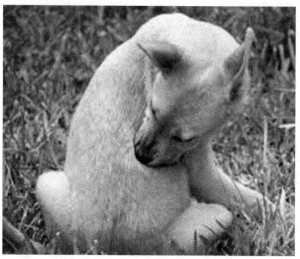

substance, like pollen, chemicals or insect saliva, as a threat and responds by increasing the production of histamines in the dog's systems.

A lot of dogs suffer from itchy skin.

Cheeks, belly, feet, the armpit region and ears are commonly affected. Allergies can develop over months or years as your dog becomes sensitized to certain foods, pollens, molds, or dyes. Common environmental allergens include fleas, dust mites, mold, and pollen. Common food allergens are fish, beef, chicken, and soy.

Dogs with skin allergies lick, chew, and scratch profusely. Golden Retrievers and German Shepherd are especially prone to allergies. Allergies can develop into a chronic inflammatory disease called atopic dermatitis, which can worsen during certain seasons such as Spring when there is a lot of pollen in the air.

Irritant Contact Dermatitis

Unlike atopic dermatitis, this type of allergy happens suddenly when your dog comes into contact with a substance triggers an immediate skin reaction, such as by touching road salt, poison ivy, detergents, acids or other chemicals. Such skin reactions tend to appear in places that have less fur cover, like the foot pads, belly, and nose. Ulcers, blisters or red bumps are signs of a skin reaction. Treatment includes preventing the dog from being exposed to the dangerous substance again.

Another skin condition is *reoccurring bacterial dermatitis* gives your dog patches of hair loss that appear to be red crusted, scaly skin, with tiny inflamed blisters that turn into additional crusty skin.

Malassezia infections—yeast infection—is a chronic skin condition. These infections are more common in wheat highland white terriers, and cocker spaniels. Malassezia causes greasy skin that gives off odor. When there is fungi or yeast you often see round, pale spots with scaly edges.

Treating Allergies with CBD

Skin allergies can be treated but not cured. Often treatment is allergy medication, such as corticosteroids like Prednisone, antihistamines like benadryl, and cyclosporine like Atopica. Other times your vet may prescribe a vaccine in the hopes of reducing the symptoms over time. Thirdly, various topicals, like shampoos and conditioners, are used to reduce symptoms of dermatitis.

Shirley's Husky/Chow mix, Charlie, licked his paw so excessively that the paw was bald. Shirley inspected the paw to see what was causing the irritation and cleaned it. The paw was red and chapped from the constant licking. Shirley could do nothing to stop Charlie from his constant licking. Even the Queen Anne color failed because Charlie still chewed his bandages off.

A friend suggested that Shirley try using cannabis. Shirley rubbed the coconut oil-based topical CBD into the skin on Charlie's hairless paw. While Charlie continued licking his paw, Shirley was encouraged when, in less than 24 hours, the redness subsided. She applied CBD to Charlie's twice a day. In less than a week, Charlie stopped licking and the fur began growing back.

If your dog habitually licks itself, cannabis oil may help. Clean the "hot" spot with warm water and rub a topical CBD like coconut-infused cannabis oil into the skin. Both cannabinoids and coconut oil have anti-bacterial qualities to help soothe your dog's skin. For best results, remove the fur— shave it if needed—to expose the skin, then rub cannabis oil liberally into the skin in the affected area. Allow 10 to 15 minutes for the topical to penetrate the skin. Feed your dog right after applying the cream or spray to distract them and stop them from licking/scratching the area. Remember to use hemp-based products, which are free of THC, which is not good for dogs.

Research has shown that use of hemp seed oil increases essential fatty acids in the skin. It is believed that high amount of omega-6 and omega-3 polyunsaturated fatty acids in the oil is what relieves the symptoms of atopic dermatitis. Topicals balms and sprays containing CBD, as well as other compounds like aloe vera, honey, and coconut oil can be applied directly to your dog's skin. Topical are great for treating itchy areas and wounds caused by excessive biting, scratching, or licking.

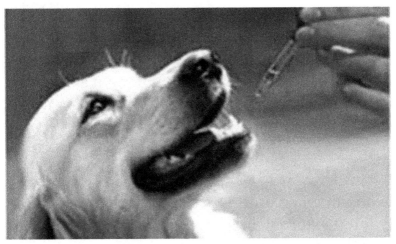

Hemp-based CBD can help soothe itchy skin.

Always follow the instructions on the package. Monitor your dog's reaction, and adjust the dose as needed. It can help to distract your dog after applying the spray or cream by giving it a snack or chew toy to stop it from licking away the soothing oil.

CBD oil has also been shown to promote healthy skin growth. Different products should be used for different issues. For example, while CBD can treat many common skin problems, only CBG and CBCa work with fungal infections, which are exacerbated by low fatty acids in low protein diets. If your dog suffers from something like ringworm, a full-spectrum CBD extract that includes CBG or CBCa or both should be used. Topical cannabis products made with oil are recommended for dandruff and flaky skin over those made with alcohol, because alcohol tends to dry out the skin.

CBD can be added to home remedies such as oatmeal baths to reduce itching and inflammation, yogurt snacks to prevent yeast infections, a cool chamomile tea spray, an Epsom salt bath to help heal open sores, and eucalyptus spray to soothe the skin.

Parasites

When dogs go outdoors they can pick up unwanted external and internal parasites. However, even indoor dogs can become hosts to parasites tracked indoors by humans and other pets. One

flea can start a popula-
tion that can infest an
entire house. *Dermatitis
Alopecia* is a common skin
condition caused by fleas,
mites and other parasites.
Sarcoptic mange is caused
by tiny mites that burrow
through a dog's skin, causing pain
and itching.

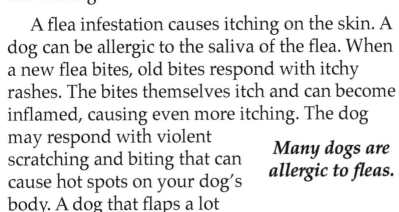

A flea infestation causes itching on the skin. A
dog can be allergic to the saliva of the flea. When
a new flea bites, old bites respond with itchy
rashes. The bites themselves itch and can become
inflamed, causing even more itching. The dog
may respond with violent
scratching and biting that can
cause hot spots on your dog's
body. A dog that flaps a lot

**Many dogs are
allergic to fleas.**

with his ears can suffer from ear mites. Especially
black earwax indicates the presence of ear mites.

Obviously, the first course of action is to get
rid of the parasites feasting upon your dog. This
may be with a flea bath, or application of flea-kill-
ing substance, or alternatively by ingestion of a
chewable pharmaceutical like NexGard®—which
requires a vets prescription, and kills fleas and
tick internally.

After the parasites have been eradicated, the
next action is to soothe and heal the bites and

resulting inflammation. A CBD-based topical or spray is and excellent option because of CBD's anti-inflammatory actions.

Hormonal Imbalances

Hormonal imbalances caused by organ disease can cause itchy, dry skin or hair loss in dogs. Sudden hair loss, weight loss, change in skin texture or sleep patterns should always be investigated by a vet as soon as possible. As an anti-inflammatory, CBD can relieve systemic inflammation that causes hives, blisters and whole-body itching. Used topically it can relieve itching and dry skin.

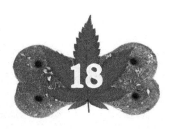

Arthritis & Stiff Joints

Arthritis is a general term for the degeneration of joint tissue caused by infection, trauma, or congenital defects. Arthritis can make it very painful to move resulting in limping, irritability, lethargy, or excessively licking the affected area. It is estimated that as many as 25% of dogs will suffer from stiff joints. Symptoms include decrease in appetite, not running and playing, lethargy, difficulty climbing stairs, pain, and stiffness, snapping or growling when touched or approached.

Osteoarthritis, also known as Degenerative Joint Disease (DJD), is caused by the degeneration of cartilage in the joint is the most common type of arthritis in dogs, especially seniors.

Cartilage is connective tissue that works as a kind of shock absorber in the joints and between bones. When cartilage deteriorates, the bones in the joint rub against each other, causing stiffness and painful movement.

Weight

As moving becomes more difficult, dogs tend to be less active to put on weight, which exacerbates their joint distress. It is important to monitor your dog's weight and use dieting and light exercise to help them stay in good shape.

While there is no cure for arthritis, there are supplements you can give to your dog to reduce inflammation and improve mobility including glucosamine, chondroitin sulfate, and vitamin E. In some cases, your veterinarian may also prescribe Metacam and Rimadyl, two non-steroidal anti-inflammatory drugs (NSAIs), both of which can cause side effects. Rimadyl can react with other meds.

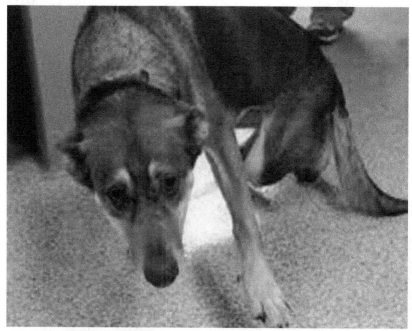

Stiff joints is common in senior dogs.

Side-Effects of Prescription Meds

- Abdominal pain
- Activity change
- Aggression
- Appetite loss
- Black, tarry or bloody stools
- Coordination issues
- Dehydration
- Diarrhea
- Jaundice
- Liver and kidney damage
- Seizures
- Skin itching
- Stomach ulcers
- Urine changes (smell, color, and frequency)
- Vomiting
- Water consumption increase
- Weight loss

As an anti-inflammatory, CBD can be beneficial in soothing arthritis pain in dogs, as a daily supplement for on-going support as well as a spot-treatment for localized relief. When using topically, be sure the affected area is shaven and clean. Apply CBD oil or tincture to the area and rub it thoroughly until absorbed into the skin. Keep your dog restrained for at least 10 minutes to keep it from licking the CBD away.

The exact dose your dog needs will depend on condition, their breed and size, and the strength of the supplement you're using. When using CBD oil, for example, generally stick to doses of roughly 2-4 drops of oil administered 2-4 times daily.

Hip Dysplasia

Hip dysplasia is an abnormal formation of the hip socket that, in its severe form, can cause crippling lameness and painful arthritis of the joints. It is a genetic trait that is affected by environmental factors. This condition is caused by a misalignment in the formation of the hip joint. Signs and symptoms include acute pain in the hip as well as the development of a limp.

According to doctors who have prescribed medication for hip dysplasia, CBD oil reduces the pain. It also reduces inflammation, which many medications cannot do.

In a healthy dog, the head of the femur will fit tightly into the socket of the pelvis. Dogs with hip dysplasia, however, have malformed joints in which the bones grind against each other.

They'll usually have a deformed femoral head, as well as a shallow hip socket. This causes abnormally fast wear-and-tear of the hip joint and will usually lead to lameness and arthritis later on.

If your dog suffers from hip dysplasia, you might also see them struggling to get up and lay down. The abnormal friction caused by the poorly formed joint causes severe pain and chronic inflammation, especially after exercising. In order to try and reduce this pain, your dog will usually try to move the affected hip as little as possible.

Hip dysplasia is sometimes corrected with surgery. depend on the animal's age and overall health, as well as the severity of their condition and your financial considerations.

Blake Armstrong's dog Rosie suffered from hip dysplasia. Rosie was lazy, lethargic and struggled just to get up or lay down. She became inactive

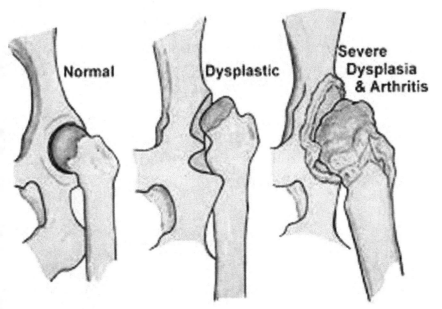

Hip dysplasia is a painful condition where the hip joint does not fit properly into the join.

and lost interest in going on walks, playing fetch, or any other kind of physical activity. Because Rosie was so inactive, Blake had difficulty keeping her weight in check.

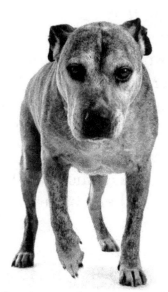

Seniors often struggle with joint stiffness.

Blake, who provides pet product reviews and helpful information about dogs on his site, *Cannabis for Pets*, turned Rosie's condition around almost entirely with CBD. A combination of CBD oil, treats, and a topical balm, reduced the inflammation in Rosie's hip in a matter of weeks. As the inflammation in her hip was relieved, Rosie regained her strength and was herself again.m, reduced the inflammation in Rosie's hip in a matter of weeks. As the inflammation in her hip was relieved, Rosie regained her strength and was herself again.

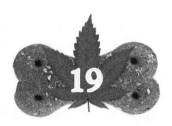

19

Epilepsy & Seizures

Seizures are a common symptom of neurological conditions affecting the brain, spinal cord, and nervous system. Conditions such as epilepsy, affect the proper functioning of neurons. A seizure is an involuntary disturbance of the brain that causes muscle spasms. During a seizure, your dog's muscles contract uncontrollably, then relax with a twitching motion.

Epilepsy is a neurological disorder that causes dogs to have recurring seizures through out their lives, often called "convulsions" or "fits."

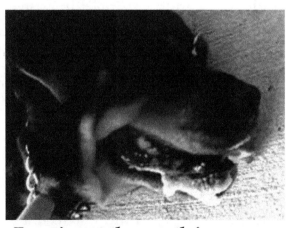

Foaming at the mouth is common during a seizure.

A seizure is an involuntary Some seizures
disturbance of the brain that are subtle, causing
causes muscle spasms. symptoms such as
staring, hyperven-
tilating, and rapid eye movements or blinking.
Other seizures can be more severe, causing un-
controllable physical fits, shaking, tremors, and
sometimes even a complete loss of consciousness.

Symptoms accompanying a seizure include
collapsing, extending the limbs out wide, jerking
or twitching of the muscles, loosing consciousness, chewing or biting the air, barking and whin-
ing, loss of bowel/bladder control, drooling,
appearing dazed or confused, and foaming of the
mouth. While these symptoms are natural, it is
hard to not be frightened by them. Keep calm and
wait the out the seizure.

Some breeds, for example, are more prone
to develop epilepsy, including Beagles, Cocker
Spaniels, German Shepherds, Siberian Huskies,
and Bernese Mountain Dogs. Seizures can be
triggered by injury, inconsistent blood pressure,
electrolyte imbalances, food poisoning, or brain
cancer.

Treating Seizures with CBD

CBD is highly-regarded for its strong anticonvul-
sant properties. Emilio Perucca, Professor at the
University of Pavia and Director of the Clinical

Trial Center of the C. Mondino National Neurological Institute in Pavia, demonstrated that CBD can reduce the frequency and severity of seizures in humans. The American Epilepsy Society has officially confirmed that CBD helps reduce epileptic seizures.

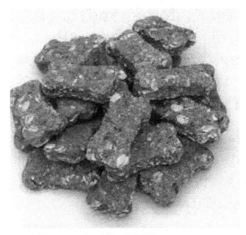

Dogs love CBD treats.

How exactly CBD works to control seizures, however, isn't clear. Some research suggests that, once processed by the Endocannabinoid System, CBD has the ability to affect specific receptors and channels in the brain to help calm the rapid, abnormal firing of neurons, and thereby help control seizures.

Unlike many pharmaceutical medicines prescribed for seizures, CBD produces few serious side effects. The only side effects dog owners have reported after using CBD is some slight temporary drowsiness.

You may give your dog 1-2 drops of CBD tincture or oil after the seizure has subsided. Seizures tend to cause disorientation and a loss of balance,

before, during, and/or after the seizure itself.
CBD can help reduce the severity of these symptoms and the likelihood of their reoccurring.

Cautions

During a seizure, stay away from your dog's
mouth because it may bite you. If at risk of injury,
such as by falling down the stairs, move your dog
slightly to protect it.

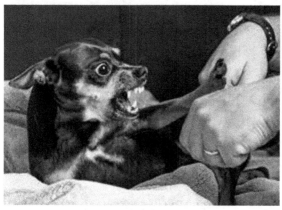

**Your dog may bite you
during a seizure.**

Your dog's
seizure will
last a few
seconds to
a few min-
utes. Keep a
record of the
time and the
duration of
seizures for
your veteri-
narian who
will want
this information. If a seizure lasts more than five
minutes, contact your veterinarian immediately
because the longer your dog seizes, the longer its
body temperature will remain dangerously high.

Using CBD Oil for Epilepsy

CBD oils are best administered as drops under
your dog's tongue, which ensures the fastest

relief from symptoms. The exact dose for your dog will vary depending on its breed and condition, as well as the brand of oil you're using. Generally, the recommended dose of CBD

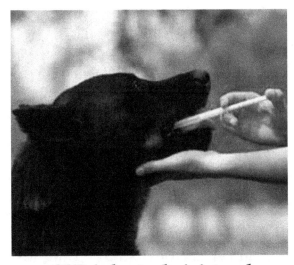

CBD is best administered sublinqually—under the tongue.

oil for dogs is roughly 2-4 drops taken 2-4 times daily.

Some dogs hate the taste of CBD and resist having it put under their tongue. If you have trouble administering CBD oil to your dog, experiment with CBD capsules or treats instead. Capsules are easier to hide in a treat or food. CBD treats are formulated to mask the flavor of the CBD and can be given to your dog on their own who is likely to scarf it down.

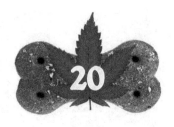

20

Cancer & Tumors

Cancer is a devastating diagnosis. Cancer is the leading cause of death among dogs, with estimates that 50% of dogs over 10 years old will develop cancer.

Cancer is a characterized by the abnormal growth of cells in various parts of the body. These abnormal cells grow uncontrollably and, over time, begin destroying body tissue and hinder the body's ability to function properly.

Whereas healthy cells constantly grow, multiply, then die off—a process called "apoptosis" or programmed cell death—cancer cells are not programmed to die and instead continually produce cancerous cells, which may—when malignant—or may not—when benign—spread to other areas of the body.

Cancer is not a single disease, rather it is a wide variety of diseases, all of which spread and affect the body differently. We tend to immediately think of cancer as terminal, but many cases are treatable and some cancers are benign.

Chemo Different for Dogs

There is a major difference between human and veterinary chemotherapy. Veterinary chemotherapy is inherently designed to be palliative, while chemotherapy for humans is designed to be a treatment to effectively cure the condition. In other words, veterinary chemo is less intrusive, with the goal to improve your dog's well-being while minimizing side effects.

CBD is an effective palliative for treating the symptoms of chemo, including managing pain and inflammation as well as help to curb gastrointestinal symptoms like vomiting and nausea. In doing so, CBD can also indirectly help animals and humans gain back their appetite, which they may lose due to their cancer or treatment.

Researchers Chakravarti, Ravi and Ganja demonstrated in 2014 that regular doses of cannabis oil reduce can kill cancerous tumors without damaging the surrounding tissue. This happens as a result of CBD's ability to regulate inter-and intracellular communication. When CBD interacts with CB receptors on the surface of cancer cells, it encourages them to "stick" to white blood cells, which eventually results in their destruction.

How Cannabinoids Kill Cancer

- ## Anti-proliferative
  Halts growth of cancer cells

- ## Anti-metastatic
  Prevents spread of cancer

- ## Anti-angiogenic
  Prevents growth of new blood
  vessels to feed tumor

- ## Pro-apoptotic
  Provokes cancer cells to self-destruct

Ceramide

When THC connects to the CB1 and CB2 cannabinoid receptor site on the cancer cell, it induces an increase in ceramide synthesis, which leads to the cancer cell's death. A normal cell does not produce ceramide when it is near THC, and is thusly not affected by THC.

The key to the cancer killing process is the accumulation of ceramide in the system. This means that by taking CBD and THC, at a steady rate over a period of time, the patient will keep metabolic pressure on the cancer cell death pathway. There are commercially available cannabinoids, such as *dronabinol* and *nabilone*, are approved drugs for the treatment of cancer-related side effects in human, like fatigue, pain, nausea, vomiting, decreased blood cell count, hair loss, and mouth sores. Consult your vet about the availability of these cannabinoids for dogs.

Administering CBD

For best results, when treating your dog's cancer with cannabis, start low and slowly increase to double the recommended dose, administered three to four times daily instead of twice.

Hemp-based CBD is safe for dogs because of its low THC content. However, administering THC—using cautions made by Dr. Gary Richter about dosing because of THC's above-described impact upon ceramide synthesis and resulting cancer cell death. Your veterinarian may also prescribe pharmaceutical medications to help your dog be more comfortable but such treatment can get pricy and result in extreme lethargy.

Monitor your dog's progress no matter which medications it is consuming and track all observations in a journal.

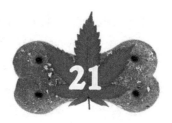

21

Living & Aging Well

CBD as an herbal supplement can help dogs live a happier, healthier, and more pain-free lives. CBD's healing properties result from its action on the endocannabinoid system, which is present throughout your dog's body. When the endocannabinoid system functions properly, your dog's body is better able to maintain a state of balance and homeostasis.

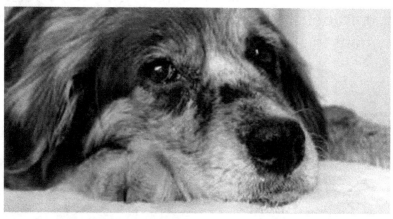

CBD is an effective immune booster for senior dogs.

Most researchers and animal experts agree that there are no significant adverse side effects from using CBD. For most dogs, CBD oil in small doses is calming; however for other dogs, CBD may work as a mild stimulant over short periods. While this may seem a paradoxical reaction it is how the endocannabinoid system maintains balance and an harmonious state.

Prevention is always the best medicine.

General Immune Support

However, in contrast to the common veterinary point of view to prescribe 'drugs first', dog owners tend to believe good preventive care involves being pro-active in their dog's well-being with proper exercise, and nutrition, along with adequate play workouts that best suits their dog—in addition to annual veterinary checkups.

The typical traditional one-size-fits-all approach to canine health has significant limitations and may do more harm than good. This is especially distressing when safe alternative options like CBD are available but not discussed by vets with dog owners and may even be dismissed without consideration.

Proactive integrative medicine looks to identity health issues before disease occurs and promotes wellness with lifestyle choices, which is opposite of much of the reactive medical dog care approach. Prevention is always the best medicine.

CBD as a daily dietary supplement can be looked upon as an integral part of keeping your dog's basic physiology and emotional makeup in top condition.

In addition to supplementing your dog's diet with CBD, the key to creating a balanced endocannabinoid system are to avoid excessive prescription of drugs like antibiotics, steroids, chemical pest repellents and parasite preventives. The more toxins that build up in your dog's body, the less effective the immune system is and the more likely your dog will struggle with age related inflammatory conditions.

This is especially important if your dog is a senior who getting up in years. Dogs are very good at hiding illness and pain, so don't wait until there seems to be a problem to intervene.

Senior Canines

Many dog owners have reported using CBD to provide palliative—treat-but-not-cure, care for their older, mature dogs with great success. They say that quality of their dog's life vastly improved after using CBD. Older dogs given CBD are often described as having reverted back their once youthful vigorous, vital selves. Senior dogs consuming CBD on a daily basis seemed especially happier; slept better, had more appetite and gained back essential body weight. Elder dogs showed increased energy, had more stamina and endurance and were, overall, more contented in their later years.

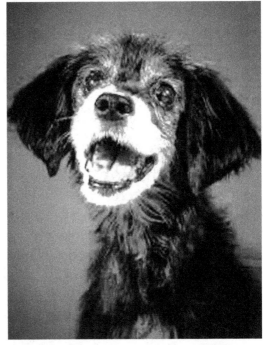

Senior dogs consuming CBD on a daily basis seem happier.

Importantly, dogs given CBD seemed more playful, lively and sociable, having regained the ability to move about freely. Appreciative dog owners agree that CBD can be the elixir of life for their beloved senior dogs.

Health Conditions of Aging

Aging in dogs is usually accompanied by a variety of health conditions. Large breed dogs tend to age at a faster rate than do smaller dogs. Symptoms of aging in dogs includes clouded eyes and vision loss, bad breath, urinating issues, lumps and skin problems, bloody gums, weight fluctuation, mobility issues, non-responsiveness, and behavioral problems.

Bad Breath

Bad breath—halitosis—is caused by a build-up of bad-smelling bacteria in the mouth, throat or gut. The first mode of action is to give the teeth and gums a good scrubbing with doggie toothpaste or treats specially designed to clean teeth. However, persistent foul-smelling breath may be a sign of something worse such as a dental, gastrointestinal, or respiratory infections.

CBD treats can help quell your dog's bad breath by helping to keep the teeth cleaned while addressing bacterial infections internally. Recom-

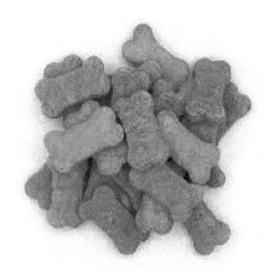

CBD cookies remove plaque as your dog chews the treat.

mended are the hard "cookie" type treats because they remove plaque from the teeth while chewing. Disney's breath was not pleasant. I bought a pack of cannabis treats in the pet store and gave Disney one a day. In 3 days her breath was nice and sweet!!! High-quality hard chew toys can help give your dog's teeth a good scrub. Foods like yogurt, brown rice, carrots, parsley and coconut oil can help improve digestion.

Urination Issues

The list of causes of urinary problems—infrequent or incontinent—in dogs is extensive, from stress to cancer or even debris in the urethra. Of course, not all of these issues can be treated with cannabis, many can. CBD has strong anti-inflammatory action. Reducing inflammation soothes associated pain, making it helpful for conditions like urinary tract infections, bladder inflammation or dehydration.

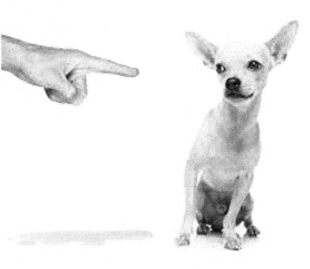

Urinary incontinence occurs

CBD oil may help reduce incontinence.

when a house-trained dog pees indoors. It may be minor leakage or full bladder expulsion but either way, it is an unhygenic mess. There are many causes for urinary incontinence in dogs that require veterinarian diagnosis—such as hormone imbalances, spinal injury, prostate disorders, weak bladder or sphincter muscles, and urinary tract infections, for example. CBD supplements can help. Giving your dog CBD oil, tincture, or dog treats twice daily can help, especially to soothe chronic pain that accompanies such degenerative disorders.

The number of "accidents" can be reduced by taking your dog out more often—every hour if necessary—combined with using rewards when peeing outside. Shirley who had problems with her little Raven peeing in the house. In response, Shirley watched Raven closely for a few days, scolding her when looking as if she were about to pee inside and then taking her out immediately, where she calmly encouraged Raven to pee and rewarded her with "Good, Girl!" and a treat when peeing. Shirley also took Raven out for more frequent walks and limited her assess to water after 8:00 pm.

Eye problems

Eye problems can make getting through daily life difficult and uncomfortable, no matter what the cause. Whether its allergies causing itching, red-

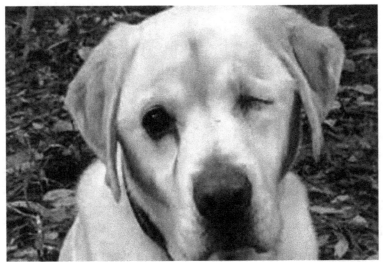

Senior dogs can suffer a number of eye problems.

ness and excessive tearing or other, more serious issues like glaucoma, cataracts, or Progressive Retinal Atrophy, which causes degeneration of retinal tissue, your dog's eye problems can be uncomfortable and may pose mobility issues, as well.

Conjunctivitis—pink eye—is common in dogs. Puffy eye lid is another symptom. Conjunctivitis is painful and irritating. You can boost your dog's immunity to fight it with CBD oil for dogs, which has been shown to decrease susceptibility to infectious diseases.

Because CBD improves immune functions and reduces susceptibility to infection, regular therapeutic administration of CBD tinctures and treats can help reduce the likelihood of developing eye problems.

Dragging Butt on the Ground

It can be amusing when your dog scoots its bottom on the ground, but chances are, it's because your canine friend is uncomfortable. Unless the cause is obvious, like a dangling turd, the distress is likely due to inflammation or parasitic irritation around the anus.

Applying a warm compress on the anus to help relieve immediate pain should be the first mode of action to reduce swelling or straining of the rectum. Increasing fiber in your dog's diet can be helpful. CBD oil rubbed into the area around the anus can help reduce swelling and potentially reduce parasitic infestation. Hemp-based CBD

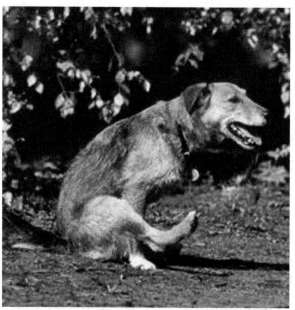

in coconut oils that is absorb directly into the bloodstream is recommended.

If warm compresses and CBD don't remedy the problem in a few days, take your dog to

Dragging the butt may be sign of inflammed anus.

your veterinarian for a check up and advice. The vet may want to test your dog for allergies or infections and examine it for more serious issues like a tumor.

Loss of Balance

Watching your pooch struggle to maintain balance can be disheartening. Unless you know the cause, such as a recent bump to the head or a powerful pain medication, for example, watching your dog fall or struggle to walk is worrisome. A chronic loss of balance is almost always an indication of a bigger problem. Though it could be something as simple as an ear infection, canine loss of balance can be a symptom of brain swelling due to traumatic injury, a tumor on the brain, or a dangerous infection. While CBD oil supplementation may help reduce or prevent damage to the brain, your

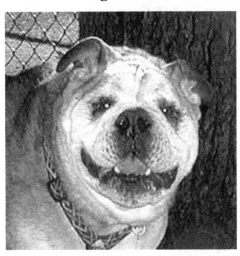

Seniors often have mobility issues.

dog's loss of balance should always be addressed by a veterinarian.

Abnormal Heart Rate

Always take an elevated or abnormal heart rate seriously. While the cause of abnormally heart rate can result from a relatively simple issue like anxiety or strenuous exercise, a more concerning cause could be at work, such as heart disease and pending congestive heart failure.

There is ample research outlining the dangers of cannabis consumption by a dog with a weak heart, the caution is for THC, not CBD. In fact, recent research by Walsh et al. suggests CBD may actually help protect the heart and prevent it from future failure. To gain the benefits of CBD for heart health, administer supplements or tinctures according to package instructions twice daily.

You might also double the dose for a few weeks in the wake of recovery before dropping the dose down to a maintenance amount. Additional steps you can take to ensure your dog's heart health include dietary changes and the possible use of diabetes medication.

Bibliography

Adrian Devitt-Lee / Project CBD. CBD Science: How Cannabinoids Work at the Cellular Level to Keep You Healthy. *Alternet*, Dec. 2016.

Appendino, G., Gibbons, S., Giana, A., Pagani, A., Grassi, G., Stavri, M., . . . Rahman, M. M. (2008, August). Antibacterial cannabinoids from Cannabis sativa: a structure-activity study. *J. Nat. Prod.*,2008 Aug;71(8):1427-30.

Bowler, J., 93% of Patients Prefer Cannabis Over Opioids For Managing Pain, According to New Study. www.sciencealert.com.

—Cannabis and Cannabinoids. National Cancer Institute, www.cancer.gov.

—Cannabis is an ancient folk remedy for parasitic worms! sensiseeds.com, 2016, January 26.

Chakravarti, B., Ravi, J., & Ganju, R. K. *Oncotarget*, 2014 Aug; 5(15): 5852–5872, Cannabinoids as therapeutic agents in cancer: current status and future implications.

Fitzgerald KT[1], Bronstein AC, Newquist KL. Marijuana Poisoning, *Top Companion Animal Medicine*. 2013 Feb;28(1):8-12. doi: 10.1053/j.tcam.2013.03.004.

Gallily, Ruth, Yekhtin, Zhannah, Hanus, Lumír Ondřej, Overcoming the Bell-Shaped Dose-Response of Cannabidiol by Using Cannabis Extract Enriched in Cannabidiol. ˆPharmacology & Pharmacy, Vol. 6, No 2, February 2015.

Gertsch, J., Pertwee, R. G., & Di Marzo, V. (2010, June). Phytocannabinoids beyond the Cannabis plant – do they exist?*Br. J. Pharmacol.*, Jun. 2010, 160(3): 523–529.

—*J Neurol Neurosurg Psychiatry*, Nov, 2008, 79(11):1224-9.
Gyles, C., Marijuana for Pets? *The Canadian Veterinary Journal*. Dec. 2016, 57(12): 1215–1218.

Harvey, D. J., Samara, E., & Mechoulam, R. (1991). Comparative metabolism of cannabidiol in dog, rat and man. *Pharmacology Biochemistry and Behavior*, 40(3), 523-532.

Jurkus, R., Day, H. L., Guimarães, F. S., Lee, J. L., Bertoglio, L. J., & Stevenson, C. W., Cannabidiol Regulation of Learned Fear: Implications for Treating Anxiety-Related Disorders. *Front. Pharmacol.*, 24 November 2016

Khaksar, S., & Bigdeli, M. R., Anti-excitotoxic effects of cannabidiol are partly mediated by enhancement of NCX2 and NCX3 expression in animal model of cerebral ischemia. *Eur J Pharmacol*. Jan. 2017, 794:270-279.

—Kinsey, S. G., & Cole, E. C. (2013, September 5). Acute Δ(9)-tetrahydrocannabinol blocks gastric hemorrhages induced by the nonsteroidal anti-inflammatory drug diclofenac sodium in mice. *Eur J Pharmacol*. 2013 Sep 5;715(1-3):111-6

Landa, L., Sulcova, A., & Gbelec, P. (2016). The use of cannabinoids in animals and therapeutic implications for veterinary medicine: a review. Veterinarni Medicina, 61, 2016 (3), 111-122.

—Medical cannabis and mental health: A guided systematic review. *Clinical Psychology Review*, Volume 51, February 2017, Pages 15-29

Mead, J.D. LL.M.,Alice. The legal status of cannabis (marijuana) and cannabidiol (CBD) under U.S. law. *Epilepsy & Behavior*, Volume 70, Part B, May 2017, Pages 288-291.

Medicine, C. F., Product Safety Information - Veterinary Non-Steroidal Anti-Inflammatory Drugs (NSAIDs). U.S. Department of Health and Human Services: Animal Veterinary/Safety Health.

Nichols, K. Oregon positioned for national dominance with tested products. *Hemp State Highlight*, Feb. 28, 2018.

Pini, A., Mannaioni, G., Pellegrini-Giampietro, D., Passani, M. B., Mastroianni, R., Bani, D., & Masini. The role of cannabinoids in inflammatory modulation of allergic respiratory disorders, inflammatory pain and ischemic stroke. *Current Drug Targets*, 2012 Jun;13(7):984-93.

Perucca, E. *Journal of Epilepsy Research*, v7(2); Dec. 2017.

Raichlen, D. A., Foster, A. D., Gerdeman, G. L., Seillier, A., & Giuffrida, A. Wired to run: exercise-induced endocannabinoid signaling in humans and cursorial mammals with implications for the 'runner's high'. *Journal of Experimental Biology*, 215, 1331-1336, Dec. 2012.

Ricciotti, E., & FitzGerald, G. A. (2011, May). Prostaglandins and Inflammation. *Arterioscler Thromb Vasc Biol.* 2011 May; 31(5): 986–1000.

Richter, Gary, M.S. D.V.M., *The Ultimate Pet Health Guide*, Hay House, Inc. 2017.

Robinson, R. H., Meissler, J. J., Breslow-Deckman, J. M., Gaughan, J., Adler, M. W., & Eisenstein, T. K., Cannabinoids Inhibit T-cells via Cannabinoid Receptor 2 in an In Vitro Assay for Graft Rejection, the Mixed Lymphocyte, *Journal of Neuroimmune Pharmacology*, December 2013, Volume 8, Issue 5, pp. 1239–1250.

Ross, M., Ph.D., Can Cannabis Replace ERT For Menopause? Optimizing Your Endocannabinoid System, October 4, 2015.

Russo, E. B., Cannabinoids in the management of difficult to treat pain. *Ther Clin Risk Manag.* 2008 Feb; 4(1): 245–259.

Russo, E. B., Clinical endocannabinoid deficiency (CECD): Can this concept explain therapeutic benefits of cannabis in migraine, fibromyalgia, irritable bowel syndrome and other treatment-resistant conditions? *Neuro Endocrinol Lett.* 2008 Apr. 29(2): 192-200.

Russo, E. B. ,Clinical Endocannabinoid Deficiency Reconsidered: Current Research Supports the Theory in Migraine, Fibromyalgia, Irritable Bowel, and Other Treatment-Resistant Syndromes. *Cannabis and Cannabinoid Research*, Volume 1.1, 2016.

Santos, M., Sampaio, M. R., Fernandes, N. S., & Carlini, E. A. Effects of Cannabis sativa (marihuana) on the fighting behavior of mice. *Psychopharmacologia*, November 1966, Volume 8, Issue 6. pp 437–444.

Sarchielli, Paola & Pini, Luigi & Coppola, Francesca & Rossi, Cristiana & Baldi, Antonio & Mancini, Maria & Calabresi, Paolo., Endocannabinoids in Chronic Migraine: CSF Findings Suggest a System Failure. *Neuropsychopharmacology*, 2007, 32. 1384-90.

Sasaki, K., & Shimoda, M. (2015, May). Possible drug–drug interaction in dogs and cats resulted from alteration in drug metabolism: A mini review. *J Adv Tes*. 2015 May; 6(3): 383–392.

Schurman, L. D., & Lichtman, A. H. *Frontiers in Pharmacology*, 2017; 8: 69.

Scott, Dana. Hemp for Dogs: Should You Use It? *Dogs Naturally Magazine*. April 2018

Silver, Robert, *Medical Marijuana & Your Pet: The Definitive Guide* ISBN: 978-1-4834-3734-7.

Sulak, Dustin D.O., Introduction to the Endocannabinoid System. *NORML*, norml.org.

Taylor, A., Ang, C., Bell, S., & Konje, J., Role of the endocannabinoid system in gametogenesis, implantation and early pregnancy, *Human Reproduction Update*, Volume 13, Issue 5, 1 September 2007, Pages 501–513.

Walsh, S. K., Hepburn, C. Y., Kane, K. A., & Wainwright, C. L. Acute administration of cannabidiol in vivo suppresses ischaemia-induced cardiac arrhythmias and reduces infarct size when given at reperfusion. *British Journal of Pharmacology*, 2010 Jul;160(5):1234-42.

----Warning Letters and Test Results for Cannabidiol-Related Products. FDA: US Food & Drug Administration. 2015, 2016, 2017.

___Washington state halts issuing of hemp licenses, citing budget shortfall. *Hemp Industry Daily*, December 05, 2017.

Resources

- ## Dog Products & Dosing Information
  Canna-Pet—canna-pet.com

  CBDPet—getcbdpet.com

  HolistaPet—holistapet.com

  Innovet—innovetpet.com

  King Kanine—kingkanine.com

  Pet Releaf—petreleaf.com

- ## Holistic Veternarian Listings
  American Holistic Vet Med Association
      ahvma.org/find-a-holistic-veterinarian

  Payton, Jamie DVM, University of California's Davis Veterinary Medical Teaching Hospital

  Richter, Gary, M.S. D.V.M., Montclair Veterinary Hospital and the Holistic Veterinary Care of Oakland

  Veterinary Cannabis
      veterinarycannabis.org/find-a-veterinarian.html

- ## Educational Listings
  Blake Armstrong—Cannabisforpets.com
      Blog: *Cannabis Supplements for Pets*

  Canna-Pet Ailment Guide—canna-pet.com/ailments/

  GreenCamp—greencamp.com

  GreenFlower—green-flower.com

  Hilistapet—Health conditions and ailment guide.

  Leafly—leafly.com/products/pets

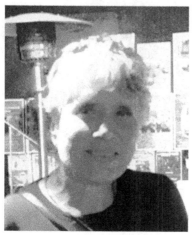

Docpotter

Beverly A. Potter, PhD ("Docpotter") earned her doctorate in counseling psychology from Stanford University and her masters in vocational rehabilitation counseling from San Francisco State University. She is a corporate trainer, public speaker and has authored numerous books on health and workplace issues like overcoming job burnout, managing yourself for excellence, high performance goal setting, mediating conflict, healing magic of cannabis, marijuana recipies (as Mary Jane Stawell), drug testing for employers and passing the test for employees. Docpotter is based in Oakland, California. Her website—docpotter.com—is packed with useful information. Please visit.

Abby Hauck is a freelance writer and founder of Cannabis Content. She writes for many popular publications including Pot Guide, CannaPages, and High Times. Visit her website at CannabisContent.net

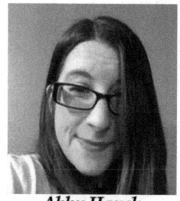

Abby Hauck

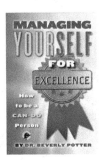
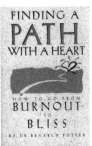
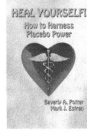
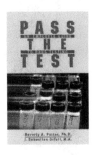
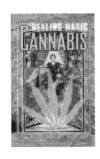
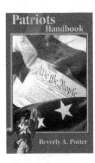
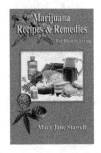
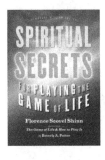
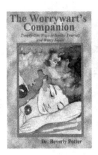
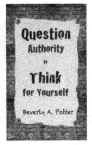
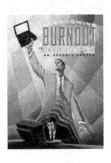
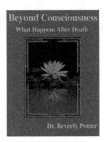
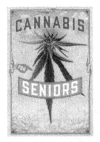
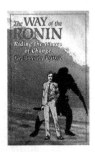
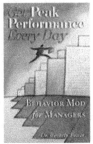

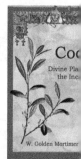
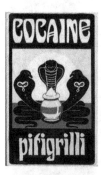
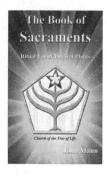
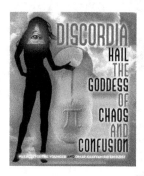
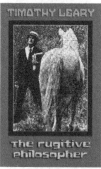
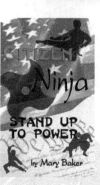
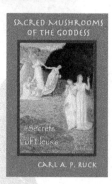
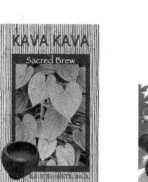
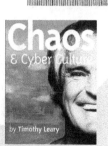

Printed in the USA
CPSIA information can be obtained
at www.ICGtesting.com
JSHW012012140824
68134JS00024B/2379